Vaccination

A Guide for Making Personal Choices

Hans-Peter Studer

GW00545172

Floris Books

Floris Books would like to thank Philip F. Incao, MD for his help in updating this revised edition.

Translated from German by Matthew Barton

Adapted by Dr Geoffrey Douch from the German, *Impfen — Grundlagen für einen persönlichen Impfentscheid* published by Stiftung für Konsumentenschutz, Berne, Switzerland

First published in 2004 by Floris Books
This revised edition published in 2010

© Stiftung für Konsumentenschutz, Berne 2000, 2001
English version © Floris Books 2004, 2010

British Library CIP Data available

ISBN 978-086315-734-9

Printed in Poland

Contents

CAUTION
The contents of this book are the result of information
available at the time of publication. Readers have to make
their own responsible decision regarding vaccination.

Foreword

The issue of vaccination poses one of the most difficult questions for any parent. Although most parents are content to follow the official recommendations, for some important questions arise. When trying to find answers to these questions, they often realize that there are no easy, straightforward answers. Although there is a multitude of available information, official recommendations and experiences, which can be helpful, they can be equally confusing or conflicting.

There is no doubt that vaccination is an important medical achievement and an effective way of preventing illness. However, questions arise; questions, which are related to views on the nature of the human being, and the significance of health and illness. At present, vaccinations are recommended and promoted around the world with the aim of eradicating infectious disease where possible. Although the World Health Organization (WHO) provides guidelines and recommendations, every country makes their own decisions about their recommended national vaccination programme. Within Europe, despite considerable agreement, the recommendations still vary regarding timing and type of vaccinations. Also the situation regarding the mandatory or voluntary status of vaccination varies. In most European countries vaccination is voluntary, except under extreme public health circumstances, but strong *recommendations* and encouragement to vaccinate do exist. For instance, research indicates that to protect against measles more than 90% of the population needs to be vaccinated in order to prevent an epidemic, and to protect those people who cannot be vaccinated for medical reasons. The ultimate aim is balance between the benefit to the public and to the individual.

This book does not intend to give you the answers you might have quietly hoped for, but hopes to provide balanced and helpful information, enabling you to make your own decision — for your personal situation and for your child.

The editor is aware of the dilemmas and questions raised, but is of the opinion that any decision taken is indeed a personal one, and that there are no right or wrong answers. It is a weighing up of risks — the risk of not vaccinating a child, leading to possible illness with potential complications, versus the risk of potential side effects of the vaccination. The issues not frequently considered are related to the potential benefits of certain infectious illnesses in childhood, be it for the personal development of the child, the development of the immune system or the possible connection with certain illnesses later in life, all of which are discussed later in the book. These relationships are difficult to quantify, in view of their complexity; research is very difficult and long-term studies would be required.

In the UK vaccinations are strongly recommended by the official guidelines and most health professionals. At the same time governmental guidelines encourage and promote more patient involvement, responsibility and joint decision-making. So, if you have any further questions regarding your child's vaccination programme, discuss these openly with your health visitor and/or doctor.

Dr Geoffrey Douch

Introduction

Making a responsible decision

Nowadays, the subject of vaccination is hotly debated, linked as it is with important questions of health and illness. It is an area where different perspectives often conflict with one other.

Primarily, illnesses are mostly viewed as dangerous, or at least troublesome and inconvenient. Vaccinations are regarded as an effective means of avoiding illness, and where possible of eradicating it altogether. Some people, in contrast, stress the usefulness of certain illnesses, and the possible risks of the vaccine.

Strident arguments either for or against vaccination can make it difficult to come to a responsible decision. Parents need to carefully weigh up the pros and cons and, where relevant, try to judge the right timing for vaccination.

This handbook offers a differentiated, critical summary of the arguments, which can help you take these decisions. It aims to help you — in consultation with your doctor — to make the right choice for yourself and your children, but it cannot and should not make the decision for you, for this is ultimately up to you. It is true that the government issues strong recommendations about vaccination, but at present in the UK there is no legal obligation to follow its guidance.

You will no doubt need some time to study this handbook, but this will be time well spent: decisions about vaccination are important matters that affect you and your family.

Vaccination in General

A Historical Overview

The history of vaccination extends over more than two hundred years, from the English country doctor, Edward Jenner, to genetically engineered vaccines.

Smallpox — a success story

Two hundred years ago, smallpox was one of the most feared diseases. At the same time the harmless 'cowpox' illness also existed, transmitted from cattle to human beings. It had already been widely noticed that milking men and maids who caught cowpox rarely fell ill with the more dangerous 'human pox.' The English country doctor, Edward Jenner, had the idea of making deliberate use of the protective effects of cowpox, by inoculating people with it who had not yet caught smallpox.

Although he had much success, this new method met with suspicion, only gradually becoming more widespread. For a long time, even doctors had difficulty with the idea of 'injecting people with poison, in order to make them sick.'[1] In 1874, however, Germany — the first country to do so —

introduced compulsory vaccination against smallpox. This
was followed by widespread vaccination campaigns in other
industrialized countries, and later in less developed countries.

These vaccinations certainly protected many people from
smallpox. However, in others they demonstrably led to
vaccination damage, or to much more severe outbreaks
of the disease, especially when people who had already
been infected were vaccinated. Their bodies had to defend
themselves simultaneously against two different pathogens. In
India, for instance, mass vaccinations in 1967 went hand-in-
hand with a severe smallpox epidemic. Only when the World
Health Organization (WHO) stopped promoting the idea of
mass vaccinations, recommending more targeted vaccination
instead and carefully isolating people with the disease, was
it possible to get rid of smallpox. Since 1977, this disease is
believed to have been eradicated worldwide, and smallpox
vaccination is therefore considered to be unnecessary.[2]

It's not all due to vaccination

Other infectious diseases, against which vaccinations were
developed, have not entirely disappeared, but have been
drastically reduced. Many advocates of vaccination ascribe
this exclusively to inoculation programmes, as in the case of
smallpox.

However, if we examine the disease and mortality statistics
that are available over long periods for England, Germany
and other countries, we can see that infectious diseases such
as tuberculosis, diphtheria, measles or whooping cough all
started to diminish before vaccinations were possible. This
was probably due to improved social factors such as nutrition,
hygiene, clean drinking water and better living conditions.[3]

Social circumstances also exert a great influence on the

spread of an illness, which was apparent from the increase in whooping cough deaths in England and Wales during the Second World War.[4]

Vaccination as widespread medical routine

Meanwhile, despite some associated negative symptoms, vaccinations have become part of routine medical treatment. In the UK there are registered vaccines to combat at least twenty diseases, and throughout the world new ones are continually appearing on the market. Some are now produced as a result of genetic engineering. In all, vaccines are currently being developed for more than seventy-five infectious diseases, and large financial investments and interests are involved in this. There are eleven childhood vaccinations at the moment as well as several other possible vaccines in Britain, including varicella, hepatitis B, tuberculosis and influenza.

At the same time, many vaccinations are now given at an ever earlier age. The UK's official vaccination programme currently makes provision for no less than nineteen vaccinations against nine different illnesses in the first two years of life. These include inoculations against diphtheria, tetanus, pertussis, Haemophilus influenza type B, meningococcal group C (meningitis), poliomyelitis, measles, mumps and rubella.

Additional vaccinations are available for specific medical circumstances. Further vaccinations are due to be added to this list, and scientists are even searching for ways to vaccinate children while still in the womb, or to develop foods containing vaccines by genetic engineering.

Many experts regard vaccination as the most effective means available to modern medicine. They believe it can be used not only to limit the spread of disease but also to eradicate it completely. Thus, the World Health Organization (WHO) had aimed to eradicate infant paralysis (polio) worldwide by the year 2000. While this did not prove possible, widespread immunization campaigns have meant that in recent years — at least in the US and many European countries — polio has rarely surfaced.

The official aim is also to eradicate less threatening illnesses as far as possible, such as whooping cough, measles, German measles (rubella) and mumps. Some countries, such as the US, have introduced what amounts to compulsory immunization. Children are only admitted to nursery and school when they can produce a certificate to show that they have been fully vaccinated against certain illnesses, which in most states are: diphtheria, polio, tetanus, whooping cough, measles, rubella (German measles) and hepatitis B. However, most states do allow exemptions from vaccination on religious or medical grounds. According to this view, it is only through a high vaccination take-up rate amongst the general population that there is any hope of eradicating an illness transmitted from one person to another (herd immunity). In the US the childhood immunization programme also includes varicella, pneumococcal vaccine, a yearly influenza injection and, in certain states, hepatitis A.

How does vaccination work?

Vaccination makes use of the immune system's astonishing defence mechanisms and memory capacity. Such a reaction is triggered by a small quantity of either weakened (attenuated, *live* vaccines) or killed viruses and bacteria (pathogens), or also inactivated bacterial toxins, which are introduced as a vaccine into the body. They are usually administered by injection. New ways of administration, such as nasal sprays are being developed.

The pathogens or toxins entering the body in this way cause the immune system to form specialized defence substances (antibodies) and defence cells.

The immune system's specialized white blood cells can memorize the surface proteins of these pathogens or pathogen-parts on a more or less long-term basis. This also gives protection against naturally occurring pathogens. If these enter the body, its defence system can deal with them quickly and successfully, so that normally the illness does not manifest itself.

For the immune system to form antibodies reliably, and for the vaccination protection to be sufficiently long lasting, especially when using vaccines no longer capable of reproducing (i.e. killed pathogens), it is necessary to vaccinate several times. To provide so-called primary immunization protection, it is normal for two to three vaccinations to be given in fairly quick succession. Subsequently, at intervals of several years, one to two booster vaccinations are given, in order to sustain immunity over a longer period. In recent times combination vaccines (several vaccines in one syringe) have increasingly been used, which are intended to immunize against several illnesses at the same time.

Unwelcome Side Effects

Vaccines have to satisfy high standards of safety and reliability. This means that they should have as few side effects as possible, and should guarantee good and long-lasting immunity. To ensure this they are subjected to animal and human trials before being officially registered. Nevertheless, vaccinations have in the past led repeatedly to unwelcome results, and so we must also examine the negative aspects of this intelligent wonder-weapon of the modern medical armoury.

Vaccines are not risk-free

The manufacture of vaccines already constitutes a considerable source of risk, since the processes involved make use of usually dangerous pathogens and pathogen constituents. Since vaccination has existed, tragic incidents resulting from unwelcome side effects have repeatedly affected individuals or groups of people, and led precisely to what vaccination was intended to prevent: severe illnesses with often permanent damage. In many cases poor quality or poorly produced vaccines were responsible for this, though the authorities and manufacturers had usually claimed beforehand that they were effective and safe.

A particularly grave example of this occurred in 1976. The American Center for Disease Control (CDC) was worried that a dangerous outbreak of influenza (swine flu) might be imminent. They produced a vaccine and organized the immunization of as many American citizens as possible. Around fifty million people had already been vaccinated before it became clear that the vaccine could lead to symptoms of paralysis. More than a thousand of those vaccinated suffered from paralysis (Guillain-Barré syndrome). The vaccination programme was halted, and the feared flu epidemic never happened.[5]

There is a fundamental problem connected with the fact that vaccines cannot actually be guaranteed to be effective or risk-free until they have first been tried out on human beings on a larger scale. However, before being registered, a vaccine is usually only tested on a relatively small research group of a few hundred to a few thousand trial participants, and over a brief observation period of several weeks.[6]

There are also many questions still to be answered about possible chemical, physical and immunological interactions which may arise in increasingly common combination vaccines containing numerous active constituents.[7]

Even when a vaccine has been rigorously tested and proven to be safe, complications can, though rarely, still arise. Each person's immune system reacts differently to the constituents it contains. We know that live vaccines, for instance, can trigger the illness they are intended to protect against in a very small number of those vaccinated. Such risks are thought to be acceptable, however, when measured against the greater risk of catching a disease by natural means and suffering from its negative effects (see sections on individual vaccines).

Problematic additives

Accompanying and added ingredients contained in vaccines represent a further problem. These are traces of substances left over from the manufacturing process. Furthermore, there are preservative and stabilizing substances, inactivating and detoxifying agents and constituents to enhance the effectiveness of the vaccines. These substances can trigger allergies and can also sometimes have toxic effects. Astonishingly, though, these side effects have never been systematically investigated.[8]

Thiomersal

Thiomersal (US *thimerosal*) is regarded as particularly problematic. It is a mercury based preservative, which has been banned in externally used disinfectants, but is still contained and authorized for use in a few dead vaccines, such as some vaccines against influenza, including the swine flu vaccine. If mercury accumulates in the body it can lead to poisoning of human organs and brain damage, as well as allergies. Official guidelines say that the levels of mercury in vaccines are within the permitted levels and are not dangerous. Manufacturers have not been asked to stop using mercury-based compounds.[9]

Pregnant women can ask to receive a thiomersal-free influenza vaccine, although if one is not available then it is recommended that the benefits of vaccination outweigh the risks of thiomersal-containing vaccines. Extensive research has also been carried out into the use of preservatives and adjuvants and there is no evidence that they are associated with any risks in pregnancy.

Until 2004 in the UK, the DTP and Hib vaccines contained thiomersal. Infants, especially those with low body weight, could receive mercury doses through multiple vaccinations. Although the levels of mercury found in infants did not exceed the World Health Organisation's safety limit, there was still an uncertain and theoretical risk. The vaccines were updated in 2004 to meet the internationally agreed aim of reducing childhood exposure to mercury wherever possible.

Aluminium compounds

Many vaccines also contain *aluminium* compounds, which chiefly serve to strengthen immune reaction. Here too one suspects that both toxic and allergic reactions may result, although official guidelines state that there are no serious health risks associated with the small quantities of aluminium in some vaccines, and that this has been demonstrated by over more than fifty years of use.[10] However, it is known that aluminium can trigger foreign body reactions such as tumour growths in the lymphatic system. Furthermore, accumulations of aluminium have been found in the brains of patients with Alzheimer's disease, but there is no evidence to date that aluminium poisoning causes Alzheimer's disease.[11]

Formaldehyde

Formaldehyde is another substance contained in many vaccines in concentrations considered to be *sub-toxic*. In higher concentrations it can cause various health hazards, including cancer and allergies.

Foreign Proteins

Then there are *foreign proteins*, which — due to official vaccination recommendations — are introduced into the young child's body with the vaccine, even though the child's immune system is only at an early stage of development. These are further potential allergy triggers. Besides the vaccine itself, impurities arising through the manufacturing process — for instance, from chicken protein — also play a role. Other additives include non-organic elements, such as adjuvants or salts, and antibiotics, such as neomycin.

The following observations must give us pause for thought. After vaccination, local 'foreign-substance' reactions become visible, for instance, as redness around the site of the injection. Even official vaccination recommendations advise careful assessment before vaccinating people known to have allergic reactions. Over the last fifty years, together with the increase in vaccinations, the incidence of allergies has risen enormously, though varying with the intensity of vaccination programmes in each country. Various studies have therefore come to the conclusion that a link between vaccination and an increase in allergies cannot be ruled out.[12] [13] [14]

Vaccinations at the wrong time

Unwelcome effects from vaccinations also arise when people are vaccinated in cases where vaccination is not really indicated.[15]

Pregnant women should not be vaccinated with live vaccines, although caution should be taken with all vaccinations in pregnancy. In contrast to the official recommendations, doctors with critical reservations about vaccination advise postponing vaccinations for children born prematurely, children born after a complicated pregnancy or birth, or children with developmental delay or difficulties. Vaccinations, particularly live vaccines, are usually inappropriate when the immune system is somehow weakened or already under stress. This is the case when a patient has to undergo radiotherapy and/ or chemotherapy or cortisone treatment, which suppress the immune system. Vaccinations can be a risk after a serious operation, as well as for older, weaker people, or those with chronic inflammatory diseases — for instance, of the intestines or the lungs (chronic bronchitis), although these conditions are an indication for vaccinations against flu and *pneumococcal* infections. For HIV-positive patients, too, the risks of vaccination must be carefully weighed against the risk of contracting an illness; for example, they should not receive BCG (tuberculosis), yellow fever and typhoid inoculations.

It is also advisable to avoid vaccination when under great stress, and during infectious illnesses such as a cold with fever. At such times too the immune system is under pressure, and already has to deal with one or more other pathogens.

It is, therefore, important not merely to adhere to the official vaccination programme, but where necessary, to postpone a vaccination after consulting your doctor. Furthermore, after carefully weighing up the risks of illness and vaccination complications, you might even come to a conscious decision against vaccination. Even if the recommended interval between *repeat* inoculations (*boosters*) in a vaccination plan is not adhered to, the effect of separate inoculations is not lost.[16] The only case where this does not apply is when the interval between the first two vaccinations giving primary immunization against diphtheria, tetanus, whooping cough, Hib or hepatitis B is a good deal longer than two months.[17]

The duration of immune-competence after initial vaccination has proved to be shorter than expected with several vaccinations (e.g. Hib, pertussis) requiring an increased number of boosters after smaller intervals, which has had an impact on the timing of the booster. At the same time there has been an increasing tendency to combine vaccinations, which results not only in the child's organism being exposed to a multitude of different vaccines at the same time, but has also led to the unavailability of single vaccines, which restrict the free choice of vaccinations.

Vaccine surveillance in the UK

The surveillance of vaccines — including their safety, efficacy and adverse reactions — is extremely important, especially as vaccines are usually given to healthy children. Before a vaccine is licensed for use it undergoes several stages of research and clinical trials. Strict safety measures apply. However, ongoing surveillance is essential as some adverse effects only come to light once a large number of people have received the vaccine.

In the UK the Yellow Card Scheme exists in order to report and collect any suspected adverse reactions as a result of vaccination. Any health professional who suspects any kind of adverse reaction to a vaccination in a child should complete a "Yellow Form" about the symptoms. This applies particularly to severe and previously unknown reactions. However, it is not compulsory and is left to the individual's initiative. Surveillance via this scheme is thus incomplete. In addition, there are surveillance methods in place linking hospital admissions/records to vaccination status.

It is also important to differentiate between short-term and long-term and temporary and permanent ill effects. A specific difficulty is to establish whether the symptom is causally linked to the vaccine. Taking all the aspects into account, long-term effects and influences on the developing child are very difficult to identify because of their complexity. As long as there is no thorough research on this subject, one cannot be totally certain about the long-term effects of any vaccination, as the evidence has been insufficient thus far.

Is vaccination damage more common than previously thought?

Research suggests that even in the case of severe vaccination damage, reports fall consistently short of the true figure. In an English study, case histories of hospital patients were compared with vaccination documents. It became clear that complications following measles vaccination, and which required hospitalization, were five times higher than had been reported by vaccinating doctors.[18]

The American Center for Disease Control (CDC) even estimates that the total figure of reported cases is at least ten times less than the actual number of vaccination complications. [19] There is evidence of a relationship between the Hib vaccination and the increased incidence of insulin-dependent diabetes in children.[20]

The great uncertainty surrounding the recording of vaccination damage is again highlighted by the example of the single measles vaccination: research literature cites the frequency with which it leads to encephalitis as being between 1:1,000,000 and 1:17,500.[21] In other words, depending on the source, such severe vaccination damage only arises once in every million people vaccinated or, alternatively, once in every 17,500 people.

In the UK claims can be made via the Vaccine Damage Payments Unit for people who have suffered severe mental or/and physical disablement of 60% or more, as a result of vaccination. If the claim is successful, the payment is not a compensation, but is designed to ease the present and future burdens of those suffering from vaccine damage. At the time of publication the amount payable was £120,000. In the US claims can be reported to the Vaccine Adverse

Event Reporting System (VAERS), which was established nationwide in the mid eighties.

In the US particularly, the question has arisen as to whether an increase in the numbers of children suffering from concentration and behavioural disorders, and even autism, as well as inflammatory bowel disease, could also be linked with early and frequent vaccinations.[22] This suspicion has meanwhile gained enormous publicity from studies undertaken by British researchers (see page 33).[23]

Vaccinations Are Not
Natural Infections

Many parents, and some doctors too, are fundamentally questioning the effects of more frequent and early vaccinations on child development. Here are some of the considerations regarding the possible influence of vaccination on the child:

Childhood disease and childhood development

Certain medical practitioners consider childhood disease to be an important factor in promoting the child's development during the first seven years of life. It is assumed that the child's development is based upon the individual influences stemming from inheritance and the environment, and that childhood diseases help the child to moderate and transform these influences. This is backed up by the experience of many parents who state that their child's attitude to life, his or her social skills, and the child's constitution have changed positively after suffering and recovering from a childhood disease such as whooping cough or measles.[24]

Furthermore, it has often been observed that the communication skills of children suffering from autism improve significantly during a high temperature, although this outcome is, unfortunately, not sustained. Doctors have observed, however, that in non-autistic children developmental progressions resulting from the effects of childhood illnesses do remain. This, therefore, indicates and supports the observation that living through feverish illnesses enables the individual to engage differently with his or her body and with the social environment.

Childhood disease and the maturation of the immune system

A child is born with what is called an inborn immune system, which is able to protect the child from birth onwards. However, from day one he or she also develops an *adaptive* immune system. This system, as the name implies, constantly adapts and learns to recognize what to defend against and what to ignore. From day one, the adaptive immune system learns to recognize individual viruses and bacteria that can make the body ill, and starts to fight them off, without attacking or fighting the cells of the body or bacteria that keep us healthy. The inborn immune system tells the adaptive immune system when to *switch on*. This process of activating the immune system is also influenced by vaccination.

Vaccinations affect the balance of the adaptive immune system, which is balanced between Th1 and Th2 reactions. Th stands for T-Helper Cells, which form part of the white blood cells. To explain how this balance works we need to look at a viral illness.

When a virus enters the body it attaches itself to the surface of a cell and injects its DNA or RNA into the cell. Subsequently, it forces the cell to create new virus cells inside the host cell by making use of the cell's own DNA (the carrier of information for personal inheritance and the next generation). When the cell is full with the new virus cells it disintegrates, and the new virus cells spread through the body infecting other cells.

Young Th0 cells can develop into Th1 or Th2 white blood cells, which spring into action to control the virus infection. Th1 cells kill bodily cells that are infected with the virus, recognizing these cells because the infected cells develop markers on their surface. Th2 cells then start to produce an antibody specific to this virus. These antibodies attack the virus on the cell surface, as well as all other free-floating virus cells in the body and bloodstream, thus stopping them from infecting other cells in the body. This helps the body to overcome the current infection, and importantly, prepares it for fighting a future infection. Suffering from measles, for example, helps the person to achieve lifelong immunity against the disease.

During the course of measles, the virus infects the lining of the eyes, causing conjunctivitis, as well as the lining of the airways, causing earache, a runny nose and a cough. Then the immune system starts to act; Th1 cells clear away the infected cells, while Th2 cells produce specific antibodies to overcome the measles virus. Usually this stage is accompanied by a fever, due to the activity of the immune system, and should be regarded as a positive response by the immune system. However, many doctors and parents are still *fever-phobic*. The confrontation of the measles virus and the immune system comes to a head when the rash appears, which is due to the effects of the Th1 response. With a vaccination this response is not achieved.

The balance between a Th1 response and a Th2 response is important for maintaining health. In particular, the adaptive immune system learns how to respond during the first six months of life, and this seems to be the most important period for establishing how the immune system will react in the future.

Numerous studies have shown that childhood infections can protect against atopic (allergic) illnesses later in life. The eldest child in the family is more likely to develop asthma than his or her younger siblings, because the older child experiences fewer coughs and colds in his or her early life than the younger siblings. However, the eldest child infects the younger ones from birth onwards!

In other words, it seems to be beneficial for a child to catch a number of coughs and colds while they are young. However, the question arises as to whether, on being vaccinated in early childhood, the developing immune system is then primed to respond more strongly in a Th2 fashion.

Vaccinations predominantly stimulate a Th2 response since the function of vaccination is to produce antibodies against disease.

One characteristic of atopic disease is the zealous production of Th2 antibodies by the immune system. Hay fever is a good example of this — the immune system produces the antibody IgE to counteract pollen but, in turn, IgE triggers the symptoms of hay fever that are dreaded by the sufferer. Perhaps vaccination should be delayed until after the first six months of life, to allow the body to come into initial contact with viruses, and react to them with a balanced Th1 *and* Th2 reaction. More and more vaccinations are being now produced and recommended. Do these increasing numbers influence the immune system more towards a Th2 response thus predisposing people to atopic illness? An international study shows that asthma, eczema and hay fever have increased considerably in the developed world when compared to countries where children are less likely to have been vaccinated. With this in mind, it is of interest that the condition we call hay fever was first described just one generation after Edward Jenner started using vaccinations.

However, medical researchers have discovered that not everything can be explained by the theory of a Th1–Th2 balance in the immune system.

For example, it does not explain why there is also a simultaneous increase in diseases that are caused by a disturbed Th1 response, such as auto-immune diseases, diabetes and cancer.[25]

Childhood disease and the promotion of health

Taking the above observations into consideration, regarding the effect of childhood disease on individual development and the maturation of the immune system, the following questions must be asked:

1. Can illness be understood as a health- and development-promoting event in the life of the individual with a ripple effect for the health of the general population?
2. What kind of research is needed to find answers to such a complex question?

The answers to these questions are fundamental in informing medical practice and patient's choice.

In recent years, medical sociologists have explored an area of research, which is increasingly becoming part of public debate, and takes human physiology (with its consequences for human development), pedagogy and therapy into account. This method has been called a *saluto-genetic approach* meaning the origin of health *(salus,* healthy; *genesis,* origin). They suggest that such a scientific approach, if promoted in the future, would help to develop research tools for the above questions of what promotes and maintains our health, which take immunological, physical, psychological, spiritual and social factors into account. How are we actually staying healthy despite daily exposure to so many illnesses?[26]

Illness can train the immune system

Fever that accompanies many infectious illnesses clearly plays a particular role in the development of the immune system. In the case of measles, scarlet fever and German measles (rubella), fever goes hand-in-hand with a transformation of proteins in the body's connective tissue: original proteins are changed in the infant's body, or excreted and replaced by new proteins typical of the child's particular age and stage of physical maturity.[27] Illness and accompanying fever also give the child the natural possibility of building up and *training* their immune system.[28] The research field of Psychoneuroimmunology clearly suggests the interdependence of psychological processes and human immunology. This provides a theoretical background to explain the common observation that children, especially infants, often gain an important experience and take a leap forward in their physical and psychological development following an illness. It has sometimes even been known for inherited complaints, such as eczema and asthma, to improve or disappear.[29] Based on twenty-five years' experience, the Munich paediatrician, Hermann Michael Stellmann wrote: 'It may sound almost heretical, but I am convinced that childhood illnesses make a child healthier in the end.'[30]

A survey in 1998 in Gloucester showed no long-term consequences of children having experienced measles, and over half of their parents noticed a positive effect as a result of measles on their child's psychological and physical development.[31]

An artificial burden with variable protection

It could be argued that the above situation is also the case with vaccinations. However, we need to remember that with vaccines — except with tetanus vaccines, oral vaccines and ones administered as a nasal spray — the path of infection is fundamentally different from a natural infection. Instead of contracting an infection through the respiratory tract or the stomach and intestines, pathogens are injected directly into the body. Thus, many of the body's own immune barriers, such as the mucous membranes or the wall of the intestines, are bypassed. The following question can be therefore raised: What impact does this bypassing have on the developing and maturing immune system? Natural infections, for example, childhood viral infections, seem to protect against the development of asthma.[32]

In contrast to a natural infection, the defence system deals with up to seven pathogens simultaneously during multiple vaccinations at two months of age — that is, tetanus, diphtheria, polio, whooping cough, meningitis C, pneumococcal disease and Haemophilus influenza. Additionally, it has to deal with vaccine additives at a time when the immune system of babies and infants is still very immature and only has a limited capacity to form antibodies reliably. Since the defence system is usually only faced with attenuated (or killed) pathogens and pathogen constituents, high temperature is usually absent. If there is a temperature reaction it is usually short lived and not high when compared to fever arising from natural diseases.

With regard to the increased incidence of allergies and asthma, the question arises whether there is a link between the artificial impact on children's immune defence systems following vaccination and a susceptibility to allergies later on in life. Generally, vaccination protection is almost always weaker and less long-lasting than that gained by the illness itself. This is the reason why booster vaccinations are recommended. Follow-up trials monitoring the long-term immune response are ongoing and awaited with great anticipation.

Breastfed babies of vaccinated mothers are less protected against infection due to the lower levels of maternal antibodies than babies of mothers who have had the natural disease. [33] However, it is also important to remember that breastfeeding may positively support the development of the baby's immune system, providing better protection against severe infectious diseases.[34] The same effect is gained for an infant by means of healthy nutrition based on natural produce, as well as regular contact with other children.

Finally, depending on the type of vaccination and the vaccine used, there is a considerable number of *primary vaccine failures,* meaning those who do not develop any immunity at all despite vaccination. As a result, people may have a false sense of security.

Likewise, someone who contracts one of the childhood illnesses as an adult will often suffer a more severe bout of the illness because of a lack of, or insufficient, vaccination protection.

Out of the frying pan into the fire?

As early as 1910, the Viennese surgeon, R. Schmidt, highlighted frequent claims by cancer patients that they had always been in good health, and had rarely suffered from feverish illnesses. [35] At the end of the 1940s, on finding repeated confirmation of this observation, he came to the conclusion that infectious diseases might offer some protection against cancer.

This idea has since been taken up by a number of scientists.[36] In controlled studies British researchers found that women fell ill less frequently with ovarian cancer if they had had mumps, measles and German measles (rubella) as children.[37]

In a controlled Swiss study of 379 cancer patients, a much lower chance of developing cancer was found in people who had suffered from childhood illnesses. The risk of cancer, apart from breast cancer, fell by 25% for each childhood illness.[38]

Similar links were discovered by various research studies on patients with multiple sclerosis (MS), a chronic illness of the central nervous system. Many of these patients had suffered from childhood illnesses relatively late or not at all. Childhood illnesses at the proper time seem to reduce the risk of contracting multiple sclerosis later on in life.[39]

Further research is urgently needed on the long-term effect of vaccinations on a child's maturing immune system, encompassing follow-up research, in order to exclude any causal links between vaccines and specific illnesses, such as inflammatory bowel disease, cancer, childhood developmental disorders (e.g. autism, ADHD), allergies and asthma.

MMR and autism

The suggestion of a link between MMR and autism has been highly debated over the past few years. MMR has been in use since the 1970s and there has been concern regarding a possible association with autism since 1998 when Dr Andrew Wakefield and colleagues published an article in *The Lancet* describing twelve children with developmental and bowel problems. Eight of the children had autism, which parents reported had started soon after receiving the MMR vaccine.

Crucially, the first signs of autism appear at around the ages of one to two years — roughly the same time as the MMR vaccine is given. Autism affects one in every thousand, and because of this time association many parents were convinced that MMR causes autism. Scientific research, which has been extensive, was unable to show any relation between the MMR vaccination and autism or inflammatory bowel disease (Crohn's disease). There was no clustering of autistic regression after the MMR vaccination. Prior to the introduction of MMR the number of reported cases of autism was increasing, and there was no sudden 'step up' in autism or a change in trend since the introduction of the MMR vaccination.[40] The Medical Research Council in the UK has reviewed all the available evidence and research and has concluded that there is no link between the MMR vaccine and autism or bowel disease.

However, Dr Wakefield and other critics have pointed to methodological flaws and bias in these researches, and they insist that the question of whether MMR vaccines can cause autism is still very much open. Barbara Loe Fisher of the US National Vaccine Information Center emphasizes that the MMR-autism question is framed too narrowly, and that it is well known, both from research and from experience with vaccine damage cases, that almost any vaccine is capable of causing an adverse neurological reaction and thus a disorder on the autism spectrum. An independent survey was carried out by Generation Rescue in the US in 2007, which involved data on around 18,000 boys and girls, and which supports this viewpoint (see www.generationrescue.org/survey.html).

Andrew Wakefield's research suggested that it might be advisable to give separate injections for measles, mumps and rubella. This caused a serious decline in the uptake rate for the MMR vaccine. Despite this, the Department of Health concluded that to give parents the choice of single vaccines would undermine public confidence in the MMR vaccine. It would also delay immunizations against rubella and mumps, leaving more children vulnerable to infection from these illnesses. Consequently, single vaccines are not part of the UK vaccination programme, they are no longer available on the NHS and no country in the world recommends giving single vaccines for measles, mumps and or rubella.

Single vaccines are, however, available in private clinics throughout the UK. It is expensive and means that the child needs two lots of three separate injections, as opposed to two separate injections, as is the case with MMR. All the vaccines used in these private clinics have been registered for use in the UK, but are not produced in the UK. However, there are different vaccines available and it is advisable to ask the clinic concerned which particular vaccines they use. In most cases clinics are happy to provide parents with detailed information on all the single vaccines they offer, including general information on effectiveness and possible side effects. As single vaccines have not formed part of the UK childhood vaccination programme since 1988, the sections on measles, mumps and rubella pertain mainly to the MMR combined vaccine.

Disrupting the Ecological Balance

Vaccinations not only have consequences for separate individuals but also for the whole general population, and we need to consider such effects carefully. This applies particularly to mass vaccination programmes, which can lead to changes and disruption in the state of equilibrium between pathogens and the body's own immune defence that took decades or even centuries to become established. This argument is frequently used, both by supporters and opponents of vaccination programmes.

Diseases are virtually impossible to eradicate

Where vaccinations against measles and other childhood illnesses have become virtually compulsory, for instance in the US, such illnesses have dwindled to a small fraction of previous figures. Nevertheless, local measles epidemics still repeatedly appear, with roughly ten times the number of severe complications than occurred before mass vaccination.[41] Similar situations also arose during a measles epidemic in Holland in 1999 and 2000.[42] Despite intensive international target settings and efforts we have only seen the eradication of one infectious disease (smallpox). But even here as mentioned before, mass vaccination only played a partial and limited roll.

The American Bacteriologist and Nobel Prize winner, Joshua Lederberg, warned that we can expect further 'great catastrophes' such as AIDS, because mass vaccinations intervene too drastically in the natural relationship between pathogens and human beings.[43]

Authorities under pressure to act

Owing to pressure from the World Health Organization (WHO) most governments feel obliged to stick firmly to the goal of achieving maximum rates of vaccination uptake, so as to eradicate diseases where possible. This, however, gives rise to various problems.

In the case of highly infectious diseases in particular, general vaccination must be sustained at such a high rate over many decades that this is hardly possible to attain without more or less compulsory measures, and in fact seems to be an illusory goal from the outset. In the case of measles for instance, at least 95% of the global population would have to be vaccinated over a period of between fifty and one hundred years if the illness were to be banished altogether.[44]

In addition, while mass vaccinations lead to the suppression of an illness, the natural protection against it, which a population develops over centuries, gradually declines. For one thing, there is less and less confrontation with naturally occurring pathogens, and for another, vaccination protection is almost invariably weaker than immunity gained through natural infection. As we saw from the example of measles outbreaks in the US, people who have been vaccinated may be less likely to catch an illness, but can suffer from a far more aggravated form of it when they do catch it.

This in turn puts the authorities under renewed pressure to act. They can start considering the refusal of entry permits to foreign nationals who have not been vaccinated against specific diseases, and can also start recommending that vaccinations be given at an earlier and earlier age. For example, the recommended age for DTP and Hib vaccinations has now been moved from three to two months of age.

Vaccinated mothers are no longer able to give their babies the same wholesome 'nest' protection against pathogens, through antibodies passed via the placenta and umbilical cord, as would be the case if they themselves had had a particular disease.

Added to this, subsequent booster vaccinations can become necessary later, in order to maintain vaccination protection. Nowadays, as childhood diseases — as a consequence of vaccination — surface more in adulthood, frequent boosters may have to be introduced to avoid potentially dangerous complications.

Mass vaccinations can also lead to what is termed a 'pathogen shift.' This means that a pathogen suppressed by vaccination can be replaced by another that, as it were, fills the gap. Indications of this have been observed in Finland, for instance, where an ambitious mass vaccination campaign succeeded in suppressing Hib infections, but they were increasingly replaced by more dangerous pneumococcal infections, which can lead to pneumonia and also meningitis, and which, in turn, required further vaccination programmes.[45] The total number of encephalitis cases has not decreased, nor have the severe long-term complications of all reported encephalitis outbreaks, despite vaccination.[46]

Furthermore, over the past few years, some doctors have observed an increase in severe febrile viral infections, often accompanied by slow recovery. The increased susceptibility of children might be linked to the absence of childhood diseases as a result of vaccination programmes. It will take time to acknowledge the increase in serious viral infections, such as influenza, as there is no obligation for doctors to report them.

Finally, we need to be aware of the fact that mass vaccination programmes are associated with compulsion and enforcement. This is clearest in the case of obligatory vaccinations. However, great pressure is also exerted when governments use advertising media to carry slogans such as 'Parents who love their children get them vaccinated,' as happened recently in Switzerland. In fact such pressure is often unjustified, and of questionable legality.[47] Those who get themselves and their children vaccinated are not simply *good* while others are *bad!* Making a personal decision about vaccination always requires careful consideration about whether it makes good sense or not, in specific and changing circumstances.

Health and illness are interlinked

Illness can lead to severe complications. Vaccinations can protect us from these and thus avoid human suffering and save on medical costs. This is an obvious argument that often leads authorities and many doctors to strongly recommend vaccination, all the more so when the official aim is to eradicate a particular illness if at all possible. The book, *Childhood Immunisation: the Facts,* may be helpful to parents wanting more information on vaccination choices.[48]

If we are to make a thorough and differentiated assessment, we should not simply set the usefulness of vaccination against the risks of an illness. The risks of vaccination also need to be considered, together with the *usefulness* of an illness. All those who have always regarded illnesses in a negative light, and sought to combat them, find this a difficult concept.

Certainly, many infectious diseases are so dangerous that it is advisable to safeguard against them, for instance, through vaccination. However, other illnesses seldom become very

serious and can even promote health. There are many
indications that childhood illnesses help the immune system
to develop in a healthy way. Other illnesses, such as influenza,
can give people the opportunity to take a few days' rest to
recuperate both physically and psychologically. However,
influenza can kill people with weaker immune systems, and it
is recommended that at-risk groups and those over sixty-five
are vaccinated annually against influenza.

Fundamental Questions

To vaccinate or not?

Whenever we consider vaccination it is important to weigh up a vaccination's usefulness and risk against the usefulness and risk of the corresponding illness. In the case of childhood illnesses, which, in first world countries, rarely lead to severe complications, it is an especially good idea to ponder this question very carefully. In cultures with low standards of nutrition and hygiene, measles, for example, has high complication and mortality rates.

The following image may help you with this decision. Imagine that you or your children wish to get to the top of a mountain. You can choose whether to walk up it or take the cable car. The cable car will get you there more easily and quickly. Walking is more tiring but offers a more intense and lasting experience, as well as invigorating physical exercise.

Both possibilities, the cable car and the walk, could involve certain dangers. How safe is the cable car? How dangerous is the path? If the path is very steep and dangerous it may be advisable to take the cable car after all. Whichever you choose, fear is a poor counsellor, for the cable car may also fail or plummet into the abyss. Trust is a better option — either in the safety of the cable car or in one's own abilities.[49]

In other words, find out as much as you can about the possible risks and side effects of a vaccination and what unwelcome, long-term consequences it could have, but also be aware of the complications and damage to health that can arise in the course of a particular illness. You may come down in favour of vaccination if, for instance, your child is exposed to a particularly high risk of infection.

In the case of childhood illnesses also ask yourself whether you have the time and capacity to nurse your child through the illness, for instance whooping cough or measles. Be clear, when making your personal decision about vaccination, that you wish the best for yourself and your child, but that there is no such thing as complete certainty. The essential question is whether you can live with the consequences of your decision, such as potential complications from either vaccinations or natural diseases. Then decide on what you yourself really want and what you believe to be the best for yourself and your child!

When and how often to vaccinate?

In the section 'Vaccinations at the wrong time' (see page 20) situations where vaccinations could either be delayed or not given at all were discussed. Read this section again before making your decision. Above all, if the person to be vaccinated is feeling ill postpone vaccination until they feel better. The effect of previous vaccinations will not be lost if you wait a bit longer.

The UK vaccination programme recommends vaccinating children against various illnesses — diphtheria, tetanus, whooping cough, Hib, polio, pneumococcal disease and meningitis C — from as early as two months. From one year onwards there are additional vaccinations against measles, mumps and German measles (rubella). A total of twenty-two vaccine doses within the first two years of life confronts the infant immune system with a large number of active pathogens and toxins, albeit attenuated or killed. In addition, problematic vaccine additives are injected into the infant's body. All this occurs at a time when both the immune and nervous systems are still developing.

One could consider not vaccinating a child so young, even though this runs counter to the official recommended vaccination programme. For many people, taking previous considerations into account, the question might arise whether the children's vaccination programme could not be individualized according to individual risk profile. For instance, if the child is going to a day nursery, the risk of the child contracting whooping cough before the age of six months is higher than for those who do not attend nursery, and could be potentially life-threatening. Take note of the recommendations for different vaccinations in the section that follows. If possible, an infant should be vaccinated in the morning, since it is then easier to notice any adverse reactions during the day.

If you initially decide not to have your child vaccinated against measles, mumps or German measles (rubella), then, if your child does not naturally contract these illnesses in the intervening period, you should reconsider these three vaccines between the age of twelve and fifteen years. The symptoms of measles are more serious when a child contracts it at a later age (see page 72). However, for girls the rubella vaccination is more important than for boys in order to protect their unborn children (see page 76).

For so-called primary immunization, most vaccinations need to be repeated. In addition, to maintain immunity, booster vaccinations are usually needed after a few years. Once more, take note of the recommendations for different vaccines in the following section.

If the option of an individual vaccination schedule were to be taken up by a large number of people there would be major obstacles to be overcome with regard to time, organization and financial management within a NHS health centre. Theoretical vaccination targets to reach 'herd immunity' may also not be achieved.

Which vaccines should be avoided?

Not all vaccines are equally safe or effective, and not all contain the same additives. Multiple vaccines, which give immunity against several illnesses at once, have the advantage of inflicting fewer problems from additives, such as aluminium, mercury or formaldehyde. On the other hand, they confront the body with several different pathogens simultaneously. Whenever possible, you should consider asking for a vaccine which only immunizes you against those illnesses that you actually wish to be protected against, and which you have not already contracted by natural means. However, it is becoming increasingly difficult to obtain single vaccinations.

Before vaccination you should discuss the advantages and disadvantages of the vaccines with your doctor, as well as the possible alternatives, so that you can make an informed decision.

What to do if complications arise?

Vaccinations trigger a defensive reaction in the body, which can lead to symptoms such as slight fever and feeling unwell. Young children can become restless following vaccination and cry or scream. At the site of injection there may be reddening of the skin or even painful swelling. If such symptoms do not disappear after a short while, or if more severe side effects occur, such as convulsions or paralysis, contact your doctor immediately. Ask your doctor to report any side effects to the Committee on Safety of Medicines via the Yellow Card Scheme (see page 22), or in the US, the Vaccine Adverse Events Reporting System (VAERS).

Some anthroposophic and homeopathic remedies can help counteract side effects of vaccination as well as symptoms of childhood diseases, but you will need to find a registered practitioner who can prescribe these (see *Further Reading* on page 109). Your own doctor might recommend treatments such as paracetamol (US Tylenol) and plenty of fluids. Many homeopathic and anthroposophic doctors do not recommend paracetamol (Tylenol) or ibuprofen after vaccination because such drugs might mask the symptoms of a vaccine adverse effect and thus confuse or delay a correct diagnosis.

Specific Vaccinations

The UK Childhood Vaccination Schedule

The following pages list and discuss vaccinations that are relevant for the UK. The aim is to provide the most important points as a basis for making a personal decision about vaccination, thus supplementing official recommendations with suggestions from patient-centred doctors who want to support freedom of choice. The schedule differs in detail from country to country. Check locally.

Diphtheria

The illness

Diphtheria is a serious illness caused by *corynebacteria diphtheria*. It is transmitted from one person to another chiefly through tiny exhaled droplets, but also via clothes and toys. The first symptoms are a severe sore throat and difficulty in swallowing. The lymph nodes in the neck swell up and the tonsils and parts of the throat are coated in a sticky, yellow-grey and strongly adhering membrane. This can lead to difficulty in breathing and even suffocation.

Symptomatic, but not always present, is a stale-sweet mouth odour.

The strain of bacteria, which excretes a poison (diphtheria toxin) is particularly dangerous. This poison can cause muscle paralysis and attack the heart muscle. In countries with poor medical care, up to a quarter of the population can die of this disease. After recovery, secondary manifestations of the disease are possible, though rare. In the UK, diphtheria is now a rare disease with only a few cases reported. In the former Soviet Union, however, there was a widespread diphtheria epidemic in 1994 with approximately 47,800 people reported ill and 1746 deaths.[50] In the UK the authorities pursue a high rate of vaccination in order to combat any possible introduction of the disease from abroad.

The vaccination

The vaccination does not protect against the diphtheria pathogen itself, but against its dangerous toxin. It consists of a dead vaccine containing the 'detoxified' toxin (toxoid) of the diphtheria bacterium. The body is thus stimulated to form defensive substances (antibodies), which, should infection occur, render the toxin harmless.

In cases of high exposure (e.g. travelling into endemic areas or nursing diphtheria patients) additional boosters should be considered. Nowadays, this vaccination can only be given in combination with tetanus as single vaccines have been withdrawn.

Since there is no single vaccine against diphtheria for young children available at present (although there is a joint vaccine with tetanus for adults and adolescents), only combination vaccinations can be given for primary immunization. This means that the child is immunized against several illnesses simultaneously. A combined vaccine against diphtheria, tetanus, pertussis (whooping cough), polio and Hib (DTaP/IPV/Hib) is offered on the childhood immunization programme in the UK, all in one injection, for babies at two months, with further injections at three and four months completing the primary course. A booster is recommended for children under the age of ten, and is usually given at pre-school age (between three and five years). This is combined again, but this time with diphtheria, whooping cough, tetanus and polio (DTaP/IPV) all in one injection.

Between the ages of thirteen and eighteen another booster is given, this time for diphtheria, tetanus and polio (Td/IPV).

Vaccination failure and side effects

The combined vaccine, compared to the no longer available single vaccine, leads to better formation of antibodies. After vaccination a slight local reddening of the skin and painful swelling can arise at the injection site, but these symptoms fade again within two days. Other common mild side effects of the DTaP/IPV/Hib vaccination are irritability, a slightly raised temperature, sickness, diarrhoea and loss of appetite. More severe reactions to this vaccination are uncommon, but the following have been experienced in between 1 and 1000 babies: a very high temperature, febrile convulsions, floppiness and being less responsive, and unusual high-pitched crying.

In the case of children who suffer from epilepsy and other diseases of the nervous system, careful consideration is needed before giving these vaccinations, although paediatricians usually advise immunization in those cases. If a child has already reacted to a vaccination with noticeable complications, no further vaccination should be given.

Children over ten years and adults are vaccinated against diphtheria with a reduced dose, since they are otherwise more likely to develop strong reactions. Following a Td/IPV vaccine, some swelling and redness may be experienced at the site of the injection, which should disappear after a few weeks. More serious side effects are uncommon, but may include: a high temperature, headaches, dizziness, nausea and vomiting, and swollen glands. As with all vaccines, there is a rare possibility that Td/IPV will cause an allergic (anaphylactic) reaction. If you think that your child has had a severe reaction any vaccine you should contact your GP or call NHS direct (in the UK).

Recommendations and considerations

The official vaccination programme for routine protective immunization recommends a total of five diphtheria vaccinations for children and young people. Three vaccinations at two, three and four months and one vaccination between the ages of three and five years give basic primary immunization. After this a booster vaccination (low dose vaccination) is recommended between the ages of thirteen and eighteen years. The first three vaccinations should be combined with vaccines against tetanus, whooping cough, Hib and polio.

To expose the infant's immune system at such an early stage to so many vaccines raises questions, which have already been discussed. Diphtheria is a potentially dangerous illness. There have been a few cases in the UK, but they have nearly all been imported by non-immunized people, mostly contracted from the Indian subcontinent. Begg and Bairay point out that imported cases have so far not led to any major outbreaks.[51] In 1994 there was one reported death of a fourteen-year-old boy who had just returned from Pakistan.

In London in 2008 there was a reported death of a child who had not been immunized.

A cautious approach to vaccination would suggest vaccinating against diphtheria — if parents so wish — only after the first year of life and in an epidemic-free period. Thus, for instance, vaccination could take place at twelve, thirteen and fourteen months of age. A booster vaccination would then be given at least three years after the last dose of the primary course, and a further vaccination at school-leaving age. Should a course of primary vaccination be interrupted, it can be resumed later; there is no need to start again. From the point of view of immune response it seems advantageous to use the combination vaccines, since these enhance the immunizing effect.

Tetanus (lock-jaw)

The illness

Unlike other illnesses, against which there are vaccinations, tetanus is not transmitted from person to person. Tetanus bacteria live everywhere — in the earth, dust, animal droppings (manure) — where they can survive for years as spores. They enter the human body through wounds, particularly deep wounds that bleed little and are contaminated with dirt. Tetanus bacteria can only reproduce well where they are not in direct contact with oxygen.

Like diphtheria bacteria, tetanus bacteria also excrete a toxic substance, which uses the nerves to reach the spinal cord and brain. The first symptoms start to manifest themselves two to fifty days after infection, starting usually in the facial area; the jaw muscles become very tense and the mouth can hardly open. Then more and more muscles start to be affected, leading to difficulties in swallowing, fever and painful muscle cramps over the whole body. Even with intensive medical care, about a third of people with severe tetanus die from it. The risk is increased in people over fifty years of age. Secondary manifestations of the disease can recur after recovery.

Thanks to good hygiene and vaccination, tetanus in now extremely rare in the UK, with an average of six cases a year since 1991. But worldwide there are about 160,000 deaths from tetanus each year.[52] This figure is gradually in decline due to increased immunization worldwide. In developing countries, largely due to poor hygiene, many newborn babies die from umbilical-cord tetanus.

Vaccinated mothers also pass on antibodies to their unborn children via the placenta, which gives them protection in the first few weeks of life at least.

The vaccination

Like the vaccination for diphtheria, the tetanus vaccination protects against the pathogen's toxin. This vaccination therefore also consists of a 'detoxified' toxin of the tetanus bacterium, which causes the body to produce antibodies.

While mass vaccinations for illnesses transmitted from person to person work by generally suppressing the appearance of a pathogen, this is not the case with tetanus. Unvaccinated people therefore do not benefit from others' vaccinations, so for tetanus there is no herd immunity.

For primary immunization several vaccinations are needed. Tetanus is included as part of the combined DTaP/ IPV/Hib, DTaP/IPV and Td/IPV vaccinations, which are recommended for babies at two, three and four months, with boosters at pre-school age and between the ages of thirteen and eighteen. See the section on diphtheria for further information (page 49).

If you are travelling to a remote area where medical services may not be accessible, and you had your last tetanus vaccine more than ten years ago, you are advised to have a booster dose (even if you have received the full five doses previously) as a precautionary measure. A booster might be required following a tetanus-prone injury — for example, puncture wounds (nail injury), wounds with a lot of dead tissue (third-degree burns), septic wounds, wounds contaminated with dirt, or wounds not treated for more than six hours. A single vaccine (TIG) is no longer available in the UK and the combined Td/IPV vaccine (tetanus, diphtheria and polio) is normally used.[54]

Vaccination failure and side effects

The tetanus vaccine gives reliable protection. Cases in which the vaccination is not effective are extremely rare. Side effects are also rare, and are largely the same as described in the section on diphtheria.

However, one can expect increased side effects when booster vaccinations are given at too short intervals. This can lead to a strong physical reaction due to 'over-vaccination,' when the antibodies already present in the body 'clump together' with the vaccine, forming an immune complex. The body reacts to this with massive inflammation. In rare cases this can lead to neuritis and convulsions.

Recommendations and considerations

Official recommendations are the same as mentioned in the section on diphtheria. It is recommended that three vaccinations be given to provide primary immunization, at two, three and four months and a further vaccination between three and five years of age, followed by a booster vaccination between thirteen and eighteen years.

A cautious approach to vaccination would suggest vaccinating against tetanus. The infection with tetanus does not leave a lifelong immunity. Even doctors who are cautious about recommending vaccination view the tetanus vaccination as very important and sensible. However, since the danger of an infant contracting this disease is normally very small below the age of one year, one could suggest waiting until children are crawling or walking outside, when the child is at greater risk of injury. There are situations in which the child might be exposed at an earlier age — for example, if they live on a farm, or in deprived social circumstances, or attend day nursery. In these circumstances earlier vaccination might be recommended.

In the case of someone without vaccination protection who sustains a tetanus-prone injury, it is also possible to provide so-called *passive immunization* with a serum (immunoglobulines, derived from human serum). This is different from a tetanus vaccine because it is made from blood. It is usually well tolerated, but in rare circumstances can lead to allergic (anaphylactic) reactions. This provides the human body with temporary antibodies to render the toxin ineffective.

Whooping cough (pertussis)

The illness

Whooping cough is highly contagious and used to be a typical childhood illness. With higher general vaccination rates amongst the population, however, it increasingly affects young people and adults rather than children. The pathogen is a bacterium, *Bordetella pertussis*, transmitted via tiny exhaled droplets.

In infants in particular this illness can be serious, even fatal in babies. It begins with a slight, dry cough lasting one to two weeks. This is followed by severe coughing fits with gasping inhalation — the 'whoop' from which the illness takes its name. A child can turn blue in the process and frequently vomits. These dramatic coughing fits can last for weeks and gradually grow less frequent and severe. The child seems healthy in between.

Babies in the first months of life can have coughing spasms followed by periods where they stop breathing (apnoea). For this reason they must be nursed round the clock. Whooping cough is rarely fatal, and death rates are less than 0.1% in the UK.[54] Complications arise in about 10% of cases, most frequently pneumonia, though on rare occasions brain damage and convulsions can occur.[55]

In adolescents and adults the illness does not usually assume such a dramatic form as in children, but tends to manifest itself as an obstinate cough. It is also possible to have the illness without any apparent symptoms. However in both cases this is problematic, since a possible risk of infection for babies may go unrecognized. After having whooping cough one has resistance to catching it again, but only for about twenty years. Cases of whooping cough are rare now in the UK due to the immunization programme.

The vaccination

The whooping cough vaccine is given as part of the DTaP/IPV/Hib vaccine, which also protects against diphtheria, tetanus, polio and Hib. The vaccine consists of an inactive version of the whooping cough infection. It causes the body to produce antibodies against the bacterium, which provide protection against infection. The vaccine is given in three separate jabs at two, three and four months, and a booster is recommended before children start school (DTaP/IPV), which also protects against diphtheria, tetanus and polio. After the first two vaccinations, protection is almost 100%. The aim is to protect young babies who are most at risk from contracting a severe form of the disease. Owing to the principle of herd immunity, younger children are also protected by the immunity of the older ones.

A single vaccine is no longer available; vaccination can only be given as a part of the combination vaccines already discussed in the section on diphtheria (see page 49).

Vaccination failure and side effects

In 1991 the new DtaP vaccine was licensed. It substituted the previously used 'whole-cell' pertussis component of the DTP vaccine with a more purified 'acellular' version, which produces fewer side effects.

The whole-cell vaccine was of great concern in the past, and had more attention than any other vaccine. Reports indicated that up to 70% of those vaccinated with DTP experienced fever and irritability. Reported side effects ranged from mild forms of pertussis infection to febrile convulsions, Guillain-Barré syndrome, cot death (US crib death or SIDS), chronic damage to the nervous system, learning difficulties and others. However, scientific research and government policies saw no proven link between the vaccination and the aforementioned illnesses and still highly recommended vaccination.[57]

The acellular vaccine has now completely replaced the whole cell vaccine, and side effects are unlikely: your baby may still experience irritability, fever or a slight swelling around the site of the injection. Overall, the new acellular vaccines seem to be far safer, although long-term records do not yet exist. Please see the section on diphtheria for further discussion of the side effects of the combined DTaP/IPV/Hib and DTaP/IPV vaccines

Recommendations and considerations

The official vaccination programme recommends primary immunization at the ages of two, three and four months, followed by booster vaccinations between three and five years.

Since the acellular vaccine seems to be safe, the Swiss Working Group for Differentiated Vaccination now recommends whooping cough vaccination in the following cases:[58]

— for children and babies in large families
— for infants who are being cared for in day nurseries and residential children's homes during their first year
— when parents do not feel able to nurse a child through the illness over several weeks.

In the case of children who suffer from epilepsy and other diseases of the nervous system, careful consideration is needed before giving the whooping cough vaccination, although paediatricians usually advise immunization in those cases. If a child has already reacted to a vaccination with noticeable complications, no further vaccination should be given.

Hib (a bacterium that can cause meningitis, epiglottitis or pneumonia)

The illness

Hib is short for the bacterium *Haemophilus influenzae type B*. In children under the age of five years it can lead to meningitis, or blocking of the throat and the airways (epiglottitis), or pneumonia. Such illnesses can take severe forms and even be fatal. Breastfed children are less likely to fall ill with this.

The Hib bacteria implant themselves in the nose-throat area of about 4% of the British population, where the immune system normally keeps them in check. They are transmitted via tiny droplets from one person to another.

Typical symptoms of Hib meningitis are fever, vomiting, headache, stiff neck and a strong reaction to noise. Subsequently, mental confusion, shivering fits and states of shock can occur. 3–5% of those affected die. The illness can be treated with antibiotics, but in approximately 8% of cases it results in deafness, cerebral palsy, convulsions or learning difficulties.[59]

Hib epiglottitis begins with swallowing difficulties and sore throat, and a high fever develops soon afterwards. The swallowing difficulties lead to saliva flow from the mouth, breathing sounds wheezy and whistling, and the voice becomes blocked and 'lumpy'. In contrast to pseudo-croup, the child does not cough. A hospital referral is needed very urgently, for there the illness can be treated and antibiotics administered.

Before vaccination for these illnesses was introduced, there were around 1600 annual infections and about sixty people a year died in the UK from Hib infections. After the vaccine was introduced, the total number of deaths in children fell to seven deaths in eight years (less than one a year).[60]

The vaccine

The Hib vaccination is given as part of the DTaP/IPV/Hib combined vaccine, which also protects against diphtheria, tetanus, polio and whooping cough. This is recommended for use at two, three and four months of age. See the section on diphtheria for further details (see page 49). A combined booster vaccine for Hib and meningitis C (Hib/MenC) is also offered at twelve months.

Vaccination failure and side effects

Over 90% of vaccinated children develop reliable protection against the Hib bacteria after the first two to three vaccinations. It contains no live bacteria and cannot cause meningitis.

This vaccination has so far proven to have few side effects, although we do not yet have long-term research. Slight side effects may appear at the injection site (swelling, reddening of the skin and pain). These usually disappear within two days, as does any slight fever. Please see the section on diphtheria for further discussion on the side effects of the combined DTaP/IPV/Hib vaccine for young infants (see page 49).

Common side effects of the Hib/Men C booster include pain, redness or swelling at injection site, mild fever, irritability, drowsiness and loss of appetite. These usually disappear within two days. Rare reported side effects include sickness, diarrhoea, allergic eczema and developing a rash. Severe complications are very rare, and it is debatable whether they are linked with vaccination. (As with other vaccinations there is a possibility that the Hib vaccination could trigger autoimmune diseases). A large-scale Finnish study produced results suggesting that 1:1700 children developed childhood diabetes as a consequence of several Hib vaccinations, and this is naturally cause for concern. The official government guidelines however deny any links between Hib vaccination and type I diabetes, quoting the same study.[61] [62]

Likewise there is concern about observations also carried out in Finland, which point to a so-called 'pathogen shift' (see section on 'Disrupting ecological balance'). In the place of the Hib pathogen, suppressed by vaccinations, an increase in severe pneumococcal illnesses was observed. Additionally, in the UK, we saw an increase in meningococcal disease in recent years, but it is anticipated that with the introduction of meningococcal vaccination (Meningitis C), pneumococcal meningitis will become the most common form of bacterial meningitis of all ages.[63]

Recommendations and considerations

In the official UK vaccination programme it is recommended that infants are vaccinated against the Hib pathogen at the ages of two, three and four months as part of the DTaP/IPV/Hib combined vaccine. A combined booster vaccine for Hib and meningitis C is also offered at around twelve months. This vaccine is not recommended for children under two months or over two years of age, as its safety and effectiveness have not been studied in these age groups.

A cautious approach would advise considering individual risk factors when deciding about this vaccination. It is proven for instance that breastfeeding provides babies with an important protection against Hib infections for the first three months of life. However, the risks of contracting Hib are greater with pregnancy complications and premature birth, and are also increased if a child attends a day nursery from an early age.[64] If a child is not vaccinated against the Hib pathogen, it is good to watch carefully for any signs of meningitis or epiglottitis, in order to be able to recognize and treat them as early as possible.

Meningitis C (MenC)

The UK differs from other European countries in being the first country to introduce the Meningitis C conjugate vaccine (in 1999). The reason for this was an overall increase in meningococcal disease during the five years prior to its introduction, especially of the group C strain.

The illness

Meningitis, meaning the inflammation of the *skins* around the brain, can be caused by a variety of factors. Most commonly meningitis is caused by an infection, either from a virus or a bacterium. Meningitis C is caused by a bacterium called Neisseria meningitides group C, also known as meningococcus. There are several groups — for example, A, B, C, Y, W–135 — and further subgroups (serotypes). In the UK, groups B and C are the most common, with group B being responsible for the majority of meningococcal infections.

The *meningococci* live in the mouth-nose-throat area of healthy human beings, especially in young adults, of whom 5–25% are carriers of the disease. The bacteria are transmitted by droplets or through direct contact with people, who are either healthy carriers or are in the early stages of the illness. The reasons for the change from carrier to sufferer are not fully understood. The incubation period varies between two and seven days and the onset of the illness can be gradual or very acute. Early symptoms often include general malaise and fever. Headache, vomiting, photophobia (the avoidance of light), neck stiffness and/or drowsiness can follow. Particular attention needs to be paid to any skin changes as a possible sign of septicaemia (blood poisoning). Typically the rash is haemorrhagic (bleeding into the skin) and does not disappear when pressure is applied to the skin. A commonly used test for this is to press a glass over an affected area of skin, which makes the rash either disappear (blanche) or persist. A *persistent* rash is a serious sign. Although meningitis is the most common presentation, in up to 20% of cases, features of another severe infection (septicaemia) are predominant.

Meningitis C is a rare but serious illness. The incidence is seasonal, peaking in the winter months. In 1998 more than 2600 cases were reported with 209 deaths. However, since the vaccine was introduced in 1999, cases have fallen dramatically.

The likelihood of catching the illness is highest in infants under the age of one, followed by children aged between one and five years. Children between the ages of six and fourteen years appear to be at the lowest risk, but the risk rises again in the fifteen to nineteen age group. Although the incidence of the disease is highest in infants under one year of age, the mortality rate is highest in the fifteen to nineteen age range. Overall mortality from all meningococcal infection is around 10% (that is 7% of people die from meningococcal meningitis and 20% die from septicaemia). Immediate treatment with antibiotics is essential and can be life-saving.[65]

The illness can lead to long-term complications, including hearing problems and limb amputations, especially following septicaemia.[66]

The vaccine

The MenC conjugate vaccine is only effective against the particular form of meningitis caused by the *meningococcus group C* organism. There is, as yet, no vaccine available against meningitis caused by the *meningococcus group B* organism, or against any viral meningitis.

A travel vaccine against meningitis groups A and C (polysaccharide vaccine) has been available for some time. However, the conjugate MenC vaccine was introduced as the immunity raised by the A and C travel vaccine only lasts for about three to five years. In addition there is a poor immune response to it in children younger than eighteen months, especially to the group C component. The Hib *(Haemophilus influenza b)* vaccine is often referred to as a meningitis vaccination. However, this meningitis is caused by a completely different bacterium (see page 58 for further details).

Although the MenC conjugate vaccine is relatively new, the constituents — the additional substances carrying the actual bacteria — have been in use for some time. They are related to the diphtheria toxin and tetanus toxoid, and are similar to those used in the Hib vaccine. This is important to know when considering the vaccine's safety. The MenC vaccine does not contain Thiomersal.

Vaccination failure and side effects

Since the introduction of the meningitis C conjugate vaccine in the UK in 1999 the incidence of the meningitis C illness has dramatically reduced. Following outbreaks of meningitis, a vaccination programme was set up in the winter of 1999/2000 to vaccinate teenagers. As a result, a

75% reduction in the expected rate of illness was reported in vaccinated fifteen to seventeen-year-olds.[67]

The reported suspected adverse reactions are considered to be rare, but surveillance of vaccine safety, failure, effectiveness and uptake is ongoing via a variety of routes, such as the Yellow Card Scheme and hospital admission records. The fact that most constituents of the vaccine are similar to other existing vaccines, which have been in use for many years, increases its safety record.

As with most vaccines, both local and general (systemic) adverse reactions are known to occur with the MenC vaccine. So far no serious side effects leading to permanent problems have been reported. Local reactions are generally more common than systemic reactions. The most common local adverse reactions are redness and swelling at the injection site (all age groups). The most common systemic adverse reactions in infants and toddlers are irritability, drowsiness, loss of appetite, sickness and diarrhoea. Older children and adults may experience headaches, muscle pain, irritability and drowsiness, and fever can affect all age groups. The rates of these systemic reactions vary with age. Seizures have also been reported as a rare side effect, although the causal relationship is uncertain.[68]

General considerations about contra-indications to vaccines also apply to the MenC vaccine, and include hypersensitivity to any constituents of the vaccine. Vaccination should be postponed during acute febrile illnesses. The vaccine should not be given during pregnancy unless under very special circumstances, when there is a high risk of developing the disease.

Recommendations and considerations

The official recommendation in the UK for MenC vaccinations is at three and four months of age, given as a separate injection, but in a different limb, at the same time as the DTaP/IPV/Hib vaccination. A booster is then offered at twelve months in combination with a Hib booster. For children aged twelve months and over, adolescents and adults, only one dose of the vaccine is needed.

General and fundamental considerations about vaccinations also apply to the MenC vaccine. Looking at short-term safety aspects, no major problems appear to have emerged so far. With regard to long-term safety we have to be more cautious, not because of suspicion about long-term problems, but because of the relative novelty of the vaccine. With the illness, meningitis C, one has to consider the severity of the illness on one hand and the low incidence of the illness on the other hand.

Polio (infant paralysis)

The illness

Polio is an infectious disease which used to appear mainly in children, but which adults can also catch. It is caused by three different types of polio virus, transmitted from person to person through fecal contamination of water or food, or from inadequate handwashing after changing nappies (US diapers) or after using the toilet.

The disease normally takes a harmless course, without symptoms. In about 5% of infected people it resembles gastric influenza with fever, headache, nausea and vomiting. In less than 1% of infected people, however, symptoms of paralysis arise in the arms and legs, or still more seldom in the respiratory muscles. In about a quarter of these cases, the paralysis is permanent. Between 2 and 10% of those suffering with paralysis die from the disease.

In an outbreak in the Netherlands in 1993, seventy-one people were involved, of which fifty-nine developed paralysis and two people died. The last case of natural polio infection in the UK was in 1982 and the last case of polio to be imported from overseas occurred in 1993. The World Health Organisation considers polio to have been eradicated from Europe, the Americas and the Western Pacific region.

The vaccination

Vaccination against polio is now carried out using an inactivated polio virus vaccine (IPV) as the part of the combined DTaP/IPV/Hib vaccination. Until recently an oral polio vaccine (OPV) had been used because the live vaccine provided better community-wide protection against polio. Now that polio has been eliminated from large parts of the world, the risk of polio being imported is extremely low. The modern IPV vaccine is considered to be safer than OPV.

The dead vaccine consists of killed polio viruses and is injected into fatty subcutaneous tissue or into a muscle. This means that defence substances are formed in the blood, but hardly in the intestinal mucous membrane.

The live vaccine has the advantage that defence substances are also formed in the intestinal mucous membrane, meaning that a wild virus entering the country from abroad cannot spread via the intestines of vaccinated people. The need for strict personal hygiene after the live vaccination must be stressed. Anyone in close contact with a recently vaccinated baby should wash their hands after changing nappies, and an immuno-compromised person should avoid contact with children with live poliomyelitis virus for four to six weeks.

Vaccination failure and side effects

Both the live and the dead vaccines give sufficient protection to 95% of those vaccinated. However 5% are either not protected after vaccination, or are inadequately protected.

Problems are rare with the oral vaccine. Sometimes it can cause mild diarrhoea, pains in the limbs and fever, or a skin rash. In very rare cases, however, the attenuated viruses of the live vaccine can mutate back into dangerous wild viruses, which can cause polio in the vaccinated person himself, or in their environment. This is chiefly the case with initial vaccinations. 1:400,000–750,000 first-dose recipients develops vaccine-polio, which leads to permanent paralysis in a third of such cases.[70] This is why, now that Polio has been eradicated in Europe, the Americas and the Western Pacific, the safer dead vaccine is used. No severe complications have so far been discovered to arise from the dead vaccine (IPV). See the section on diphtheria for further information on side effects of the combined DTaP/IPV/Hib vaccination (see page 49).

Recommendations and considerations

Official recommendations in the UK state that IPV should be given in three doses at two, three and four months of age, as part of the combined DTaP/IPV/Hib vaccination. A booster is offered between three and five years old, before starting school. This is combined again, but this time with diphtheria, whooping cough, tetanus and polio (DTaP/IPV) all in one injection.

In adults, booster vaccinations are currently only thought necessary for people at greater risk, such as travellers to epidemic regions.

In reference to the live OPV vaccine, which is no longer in common use in the UK, The Swiss Working Group for Differentiated Vaccination regards it as problematic to expose the still-developing nervous systems of children to neurotropic viruses such as the live polio virus. The group recommends vaccination with OPV only after the age of two or three years. If live vaccines are used, vaccination should, if possible, take place outside of the summer months, for its effect can be disturbed by other gastric infections, which may be more prevalent at this time of year. For the same reason, oral vaccination for people with a stomach complaint that includes diarrhoea and vomiting should be delayed until they have fully recovered.

Vaccination is important for social reasons, as epidemics are likely to reoccur if herd immunity drops.

Mumps

The illness

Mumps, together with measles, German measles (rubella), whooping cough and chicken pox, is one of the classic childhood illnesses that appeared before the introduction of vaccination programmes. This illness is caused by a virus transmitted by exhaled droplets, and lasts for about seven to ten days. Usually it takes a harmless course, and in a third of cases even has no symptoms. In a further third, non-specific, flu-like symptoms appear. Only in the last third does painful swelling of the parotid and salivary glands (in front of and below the ear and under the jaw) appear, as typical mumps symptoms. In rare cases loss of hearing can arise with partial or complete recovery. A further possible complication is inflammation of the pancreas.

Complications frequently occur in adolescents and adults. At that age there is a greater risk that mumps will lead to meningitis or encephalitis (1:400 infected children prior to introduction of vaccination). Both of these seldom take a serious course. In 20% of male adolescents and adults, inflammation of the testicles can occur, but this hardly ever results in infertility. In rare cases mumps can trigger ovarian inflammation in adolescent girls and women. Even if the illness runs its course without any symptoms, it gives lifelong immunity.

The vaccination

The vaccine against mumps consists of attenuated live viruses, and is injected into a muscle or subcutaneous fatty tissue, combined with inoculations against measles and German measles (rubella) in the MMR vaccine. Since live vaccines are involved, all single and combination vaccines against mumps, measles and German measles are free of thiomersal.

The official vaccination recommendations state that infants should be first vaccinated against mumps at around thirteen months, in combination with vaccinations against measles and German measles. Before this age it is believed that antibodies derived from the mother cancel out the vaccination's effect to some extent. The second vaccination is recommended between the ages of three and five years as part of the pre-school programme. The vaccine can also be given to adults who were not vaccinated in childhood. This vaccine must not be given during pregnancy and it is recommended that women who have the MMR vaccine should avoid getting pregnant for at least one month after vaccination.

The official aim in European countries, including Great Britain, is to eradicate this illness, as well as measles and German measles, but this requires a high rate of vaccination. Given the lack of confidence in the MMR vaccination over the past few years, the overall vaccination rate in the UK has been too low to achieve this (see section on measles, page 73).

Vaccination failure and side effects

Despite efforts to improve vaccination protection, a small number of those vaccinated do not develop, or develop too few, antibodies. In the longer term the protective effect of vaccines based particularly on the *Rubini* strain (not available in the UK) is deemed to be unsatisfactory. The recommended second vaccination seems to improve the protective effect, but it is still unclear whether protection lasts throughout life or not, since long-term studies are ongoing. However, the Jeryl Lynn strain, which is in use in the UK, has shown up to twenty-five years of long-term immunity.[72]

For approximately one in fifty vaccinated people, the vaccination can trigger 'vaccination mumps' — in other words a weaker form of the illness. This involves feeling generally unwell, with fever and a usually one-sided, painless swelling of the parotid gland (in front of and below the ear). This usually occurs about three weeks after the vaccination. In 1:1,000,000 vaccinations, a one-sided, painful swelling of the testicles can occur. There is a similarly small risk of meningitis triggered by the mumps vaccine, with fever, headache, stiff neck and vomiting. This does not become serious, though, and leaves no lasting damage.

Recommendations and considerations

As with measles and German measles (rubella), the official UK vaccination recommendation is now for the mumps vaccination to be given at around thirteen months, with a repeat vaccination at three to five years of age.

Given the small risk associated with the illness, as well as its possible usefulness for the development of the child, a cautious approach to vaccination could consider avoiding routine mumps vaccination.[73] One could also point out that mass vaccination leads to the illness shifting to a later age, into adolescence or adulthood, when there is an increased risk of complications. Studies regarding the persistence of lifelong immunity following vaccination are awaited. Caution is necessary if you have an allergy to chicken protein (egg). An allergy is present if the child has had an anaphylactic reaction to chicken protein. However, this is not a contraindication to vaccination, and should be discussed with your doctor. If the doctor decides there is a real allergy to chicken protein then the vaccine can still be given but under hospital supervision.

Measles

The illness

Like mumps, German measles (rubella) or whooping cough, measles is a classic childhood illness. The measles virus is very infectious and is transmitted via exhaled or coughed droplets. Though a high temperature often develops and the child feels unwell, the illness does not usually take a dangerous course in first world countries. The acute phase lasts for about ten days.

After an incubation period of one to three weeks, measles has an initial period lasting four days, with a raised temperature, head cold, a dry, irritable cough and red eyes. On the inside of the cheeks, the mucous membranes show fine, white dots and streaks (Koplik's spots). The fever falls but then rises again soon afterwards up to around 40°C (104°F). Febrile convulsions can occur. A reddish, blotchy rash appears on the face and behind the ears, which then spreads over the whole body. The child can be sensitive to light. After two to three days the rash starts to fade, often with the skin flaking, and the fever abates. The child now needs at least two weeks to convalesce, and subsequently has a lifelong resistance to any further measles infection.

Although the illness usually affects the child quite severely, serious complications are rare in the developed world, but measles does have a very high mortality rate in the developing world. Measles can be associated with middle-ear infection or pneumonia. However, the most serious of the measles complications is encephalitis, which is more frequent in babies and young adults. Estimates of its frequency vary between 1:1000 and 1:10,000, though the second figure is likely to be nearer the truth.[73] Out of those children suffering from measles-related encephalitis about a tenth die and a third experience lasting brain damage. There is a very small risk (1:25,000) that a late complication can develop into another, always fatal, form of encephalitis — subacute sclerosing pan-encephalitis (SSPE).[74] In recent years, one or two people in every thousand cases of reported measles infection have died from it.

Mortality rates from measles are highest in children under the age of one — a group that cannot receive the MMR vaccine — and in those who are immune-suppressed due to disease, such as leukaemia, or medical treatments, such as organ transplantation. These children can only be protected through *population protection* as a result of high vaccine uptake.[75]

Since the introduction of the measles vaccination, measles is no longer common in the UK, but does still occur in small, local epidemics.

The vaccination

In the UK the measles vaccination is given in combination with mumps and German measles in the MMR injection, using a live vaccine with attenuated viruses. At present, the first vaccination is recommended at around thirteen months of age, because antibodies against measles passed on through the mother can interfere with its effect. Antibodies can also be passed on during pregnancy. A second vaccination at three to five years of age is intended to catch children who have not responded to the first vaccination and boost their immunity.

The aim of the official vaccination campaign in the UK — set by the World Health Organization (WHO) — is to eradicate measles altogether, but to achieve this, long-term vaccination of more than 95% of the whole population is required. However, the national rate of children who have been vaccinated against measles has never exceeded 92%, and the number of cases of measles each year is constantly changing, influenced by public health scares such as the MMR-autism debate.[76] For example, between January and October 2008, there were 1049 cases reported in the UK — this first time numbers had exceeded 1000 since 1995.[77] Therefore this aim has to be viewed as fairly unrealistic.

Vaccination failure and side effects

After the first vaccination between 5 and 10% of those vaccinated do not develop any resistance to the disease.[78] The pre-school booster jab helps to increase protection, and results in less than 1% remaining at risk. In the case of vaccination failure, measles can be developed at a later age, when the risk of complications such as encephalitis is much higher.

Vaccinated mothers are also unable to pass on the same level of protection to their babies as those who have had measles.[79] This means that in the generally vaccinated American population, measles is now associated with a ten times greater risk of encephalitis than before.[80]

However, the vaccination itself is also not risk-free. The live virus can trigger 'vaccination measles' — a weaker form of the illness — in vaccinated people. In rare cases this can include febrile convulsions (1:1000) or middle-ear infections. The most serious complication from vaccination, as with the illness itself, is also encephalitis. Estimates for the probability of this vary greatly in research literature, from 1:200 to 1:5000, as a result of contracting measles itself, and less than 1:1,000,000 after vaccination. The risk of severe allergic response after the vaccination is 1:100,000.[81]

The indirect long-term effects of vaccination must also be considered (see discussion of the MMR vaccine on page 33). Measles, and the high temperatures associated with it, lead to an important transformation of proteins in the child, and can train his immune system. Several studies indicate that adults who, when children, did not contract measles and other childhood illnesses, might be more at risk of severe illnesses such as cancer, multiple sclerosis and immune-system disorders.

Recommendations and considerations

The official recommendation in the UK is to vaccinate children against measles at around thirteen months of age

— together with vaccinations against mumps and German measles (MMR). A repeat injection is then recommended between three and five years of age to catch those who did not respond the first time, and to boost existing antibody levels.

It should be taken into consideration that measles is important for the development of the immune system, and can support the psychological and spiritual development of the child.[82]

One can be concerned that mass vaccination could lead to a shift in the illness towards babies and adults, who are at greater risk from measles complications. It therefore seems best to encourage people to make their own individual decision about measles vaccination, but young people between the ages of eleven and fifteen, who have not contracted measles, should seriously consider vaccination.[83]

Pregnant women should not be vaccinated. In addition, those suffering from a feverish illness, those with a weakened immune system or an allergy to chicken protein (egg), should discuss options for vaccination further with their doctor. An egg-allergy is not a contra-indication to vaccination, but it does need further discussion (see page 71).

German measles (rubella)

The illness

German measles is a typical childhood illness which normally takes a harmless course. It is caused by a virus transmitted via small, exhaled droplets, and only lasts a few days. It gives rise to a skin rash with red spots over the whole body, and sometimes to a high though unproblematic fever. The lymph nodes behind the ears and in the neck swell up and become sensitive to pressure. Encephalitis is a serious but rare complication, mainly from adolescence onwards. In adults, German measles can also give rise to joint inflammation. After recovery from German measles, it is highly probable that a lifelong resistance to this illness will be acquired.

While German measles is harmless in children, it is dangerous for the unborn child during the first four months of pregnancy: it can result in stillbirth and malformations of the embryo leading to eye cataracts, hearing problems or complete deafness, learning disability and malformations of the heart (rubella foetal syndrome). In the UK around five children per year are born with malformations as a result of rubella, but a small increase has recently been observed, most likely owing to the fall in the vaccination rate.[84]

The vaccination

The German measles vaccine consists of attenuated live viruses, and is injected into muscle or subcutaneous fatty tissue. In children it is always combined with vaccines against measles and mumps (MMR). Although a single German measles vaccine was available until recently, this is no longer the case and the combined MMR vaccine is now used.[85]

The main aim of the rubella vaccination is to prevent rubella infections in pregnancy, as well as attempting to eradicate the illness altogether. Consequently, all children between the ages of twelve and fifteen months are offered the MMR vaccine. A second vaccination between the ages of three and five years aims to improve protection.

Given a drop in vaccination rates due to the highly-publicised debate surrounding the MMR vaccine and autism, the possibility of total eradication — as with mumps and measles — seems unrealistic.[86]

Vaccination failure and side effects

The rubella vaccine does not provide the same protection as catching the illness in the natural way. After vaccination, protection is sufficient in 97–99% of those vaccinated, but as time goes by protection diminishes. At childbearing age, no more than 80–90% of women vaccinated as children still have sufficient protection.[87] Therefore women of childbearing age should be screened for rubella antibodies to make sure that they are immune. As the single vaccination is no longer available on the NHS, women of childbearing age who are found to have reduced immunity to rubella, will receive the MMR vaccine either before pregnancy or after birth.

A possible side effect is for the vaccination viruses to trigger a weak form of the illness, which in children can sometimes lead to short-lived joint pain. One in seven vaccinated adults reacts with joint pain and inflammation, which in rare cases can continue for years as chronic arthritis or polyarthritis.

There are similar concerns about possible indirect long-term effects as with measles and mumps.

Recommendations and considerations

In accordance with the aims of the World Health Organization (WHO), the official vaccination programme in the UK now recommends vaccinating children against German measles, as well as mumps and measles (MMR), at the age of twelve to fifteen months. The vaccination should then be repeated between three and five years, so that infants who did not respond to the first vaccination can be protected, or their existing protection can be boosted.

One should point out that protection for pregnant women who were vaccinated in childhood is weaker than for those who caught the illness naturally.[88] It is therefore worth considering whether vaccination should only be given to girls between twelve and fifteen years, who have not yet caught the illness by natural means, as used to be the case. If there is any doubt, a blood test can ascertain either whether someone has had the illness, or whether previous vaccinations have taken hold. Vaccination must not be given during pregnancy. Women who were not vaccinated until adulthood should avoid getting pregnant until three months after vaccination as a precautionary measure.

One should consider the importance of experiencing a rubella infection in childhood for the immunological, psychological and spiritual development of the child.

If there is an allergy to chicken protein (egg), caution with the combination vaccination against measles, mumps and German measles (MMR) is advised. It is, however, not a contra-indication and a discussion with your doctor is recommended.

Pneumococcal disease

The illness

Pneumococcus is a bacteria, which usually causes community-acquired pneumonia and otitis media (ear infection). In addition, it can cause more serious invasive diseases, such as pneumonia, septicaemia and meningitis. In the UK, pneumonia due to *pneumococcus* is thought to occur in 1:1000 adults each year, and in some cases can result in death. Although it can affect anybody, the people most at risk are the very young and the very old, especially those who have had their spleen removed or those whose immunity is impaired. People with chronic lung or heart disease, or diabetics, are also more at risk.

All of the aforementioned illnesses caused by the *pneumococcus* bacteria are usually treated effectively by antibiotics (penicillin), although penicillin-resistant and multi-drug-resistant *pneumoccocus* bacteria have been reported. However, treatment failure with more sophisticated antibiotics is uncommon.

The Health Department considers this group of illnesses to be an important public health problem, so the pneumococcal vaccination is now included as part of the childhood immunization programme.

The vaccination

In the UK, the pneumococcal conjugate vaccine (PCV) is given alongside the combined DTaP/IPV/Hib vaccination at two months and four months of age, with a final dose at around thirteen months. It covers seven types of *pneumoccocus* bacteria. People aged sixty-five and over are routinely offered the pneumococcal polysaccharide vaccine (PPV) to protect against pneumococcal disease.

Vaccination failure and side effects

The stated aim of the vaccination campaign is to prevent infection and death. Random control trials (RCTs) of the pneumoccocal vaccine have found mixed results. One systematic review of RCTs found evidence that vaccination with currently available pneumococcal vaccines did not protect against death. It also found evidence that pneumococcal vaccine protected young, healthy adults, but not higher-risk, older adults against pneumococcal pneumonia. Subsequent RCTs found no evidence of benefit in older adults. Subgroup analysis — that is, analysis that is not age-related, but concerns other affected groups such as those without a spleen etc. — did suggest a benefit to adults at high risk of pneumonia.[98] These contradictory findings highlight the controversy surrounding the possible benefits of the vaccine.

The vaccine is normally well tolerated, but soreness and hardness at the injection site can sometimes occur, and a mild fever can also be present. However, these symptoms are usually minor and soon go away. Hypersensitivity has also been reported.

Pneumococcal vaccine should not be given during a serious illness. The vaccine is not recommended during pregnancy or in women who are breastfeeding.

Recommendations and considerations

The current official vaccination programme recommends immunization for infants at two, four and thirteen months and all adults aged sixty-five and over, as well as for people aged over two years with various risk factors, such as those without a spleen, those who have diabetes, asthma, heart, lung, liver or kidney conditions, blood disorders and immune suppression. The list is not complete as the guidelines are constantly changing. The spleen is an organ in the abdomen which sometimes is removed for a variety of reasons. It helps to protect against infection, particularly against pneumococcal infection. Those at high risk should consider the vaccination. However, we found little evidence of benefit for healthy or low-risk people. Therefore, a more cautious approach would indicate not vaccinating these people.

Cervical cancer

The illness

Cervical cancer is the second most common malignancy among women in the world and around 250,000 women die from it each year. In the UK, smear testing has led to a decrease in the number of deaths from cervical cancer. In 2006 around 1000 women died from the disease.[90] If detected in the early stages, cervical cancer can be treated and cured with surgery or radiotherapy, but the cure rate depends upon whether or not it has spread beyond the cervix.

In most cases there is no definite single cause, but the human papillomavirus (HPV) is usually present. HPV is a sexually-transmitted infection that can cause genital warts, pre-cancerous cell abnormalities in the female genital area and cervical cancer. During 2008 and 2009 the UK has seen the widespread use of new vaccines to prevent cervical cancer, which work by protecting against the human papillomavirus.

The vaccine

The HPV vaccine chosen for use by the NHS in the childhood vaccination programme (Cervarix) protects against the two strains of the human papillomavirus (16 and 18) that are responsible for approximately 70% of cervical cancer cases. Because it does not protect against all cervical cancers, girls should still have cervical screening later in life. Cervarix contains inactivated extracts from the two types of the virus. Three doses are needed: the first two are given one month apart and the third, six months later.[91]

Another vaccine (Gardasil) was also developed, which contains inactivated extracts from four different types of the human papillomavirus, including types 6 and 11 as well as 16 and 18. Types 6 and 11 are responsible for approximately 90% of genital wart cases.[101]

Vaccination failure and side effects

As this is a new vaccine, it is not known exactly how long the protective effect of the vaccine will last, and long-term assessment is ongoing. It should not be given to girls under the age of ten. Common side effects reported so far include pain, redness or swelling at the injection site, headaches, muscle pain and tiredness. Less common side effects include vomiting, diarrhoea or abdominal pain, skin reactions, fever and joint pain.

Following its intial introduction there were also isolated reports of both convulsions and paralysis. The MHRA (Medicines and Healthcare Products Regulatory Agency) said that the reported reactions did not necessarily mean they were side effects of the vaccine, and that they may have been coincidental events. They believe that the positive benefits of the vaccine far outweigh the risks.[93]

Recommendations and considerations

The HPV vaccination now forms part of the UK childhood immunization programme, and is recommended for girls aged twelve to thirteen. On its introduction in 2008 a catch-up programme was also offered for girls aged between thirteen to eighteen, but it is not offered for adults on the NHS.[94] Three injections are given over six months.

As this vaccine was newly-introduced at the time of writing, it is hard to weigh up long-term risks and benefits. As HPV is a sexually-transmitted infection, being sexually responsible will help to protect against the virus, should you not wish to go ahead with vaccination. If you have any concerns, discuss the matter further with your doctor.

Other Vaccinations

Tuberculosis (TB)

The illness

Tuberculosis is an infectious illness caused by *Myobacterium tuberculosis*, and can affect many organs, usually the lungs and bones. Specific symptoms relate to the site of the infection and are generally accompanied by fever, sweats and weight loss.

About one third of the world population is infected by *M.tuberculosis*. The organism kills more people than any other infection. The vast majority of TB deaths are in the developing world, with more than half of all deaths in Asia. The total number of deaths is rising due to population growth, but the rate is slowly declining: the global rate fell from 142:100,000 population in 2004, to 139:100,000 population in 2007.[95]

In the Western World the incidence of TB is low, but there are high-risk groups in the UK: alcoholics, HIV-positive individuals and people who are immune-suppressed, some recent immigrants and healthcare workers. Risk factors associated with this disease are poverty, overcrowding, homelessness and inadequate health services. The incidence of TB is increasing in the UK, owing to the rise in immigrants from countries with a high incidence of TB and because of the increase in people with HIV. In 2002, there were 6891 known cases in England and Wales (*Guardian*, Wednesday 24 March, 2004).

The prognosis varies widely and depends on treatment. The treatment of TB is quite lengthy and requires at least six months medication with different anti-tuberculous drugs, which must be supervised by a specialist. Compliance of patients with this lengthy treatment can be a problem. There is an increase in infection with TB bacilli that are resistant to the standard drugs used.

TB is most commonly spread through small air droplets by somebody who carries it in his sputum. It needs prolonged and close contact in order to be transmitted. In the UK about 74% of patients with TB have the respiratory form, when the lungs are affected. Other affected organs are the brain, the kidneys and bones. Specific symptoms relate to the site of the infection and are generally accompanied by fever, sweats and weight loss.

The vaccine

The BCG vaccine (Bacillus Calmette-Guerin) contains a live, attenuated strain derived from *Mycobacterium bovis*. Two preparations are available, one for infants and one for anybody else. The injection is given in the skin. Within two weeks a small swelling appears at the injection site, which changes to a papule or to a benign ulcer about 10 mm in diameter, which heals in six to twelve weeks.[96]

A tuberculin test is normally carried out before BCG immunization, that is, the Heaf or Mantoux test. This is a skin test to assess immunity to the tuberculoprotein. If there is no reaction, then the person is considered not to have had any previous contact with TB, and immunization should follow. For children up to six years of age, the Mantoux test is not normally required before the vaccine is given.

The BCG vaccine is no longer routinely given to all children, but instead the vaccination programme is targeted to high-risk groups, which include: immigrants from countries with a high prevalence of tuberculosis, as well as their children and newborn infants; people in close contact with TB sufferers; health service staff; veterinary staff; prison staff; staff of hostels for the homeless and refugees; those intending to stay in countries with a high prevalence of TB for longer than one month. Babies born into any of the above risk groups are immunized in the first three months of life.

The vaccination should not be given to patients on steroids or immuno-suppressant treatment, patients with malignant conditions, the immunologically-impaired, HIV patients, pregnant women, people with a positive skin reaction to the tuberculin test, or people suffering from a febrile or a generalized septic skin condition.[97]

Vaccination failure and side effects

The protection of the vaccine is variable. It protects 70–80% of vaccinated school children for at least fifteen years. For newborn babies the vaccine protects between 64 and 75% against general TB, and 85–100% against TB meningitis, the most severe form of the disease.

Immediate allergic or anaphylactic reactions are rarely reported, but dizziness, headache and fever have sometimes been recorded following a BCG immunization. The BCG vaccine often causes a hardened lesion around the injection site that may ulcerate. This is common and will heal over after several weeks or months, leaving a small flat scar.

Recommendations and considerations

As stated earlier, babies at risk are offered neonatal immunization, and it is recommended that certain groups of adults be immunized (see above). It is advisable to vaccinate children who are deemed to be at risk due to their ethnic background, travel destinations, or because they have been in close contact with a person suffering from TB.

Hepatitis B

The illness

Hepatitis B is a viral illness transmitted mainly via blood and sexual contact. In the case of a wound or injury it can also be transmitted via saliva. The risk of contracting Hepatitis B from close household contacts (probably through saliva) is low but possible. The virus passes through the blood to the liver where it can lead to liver inflammation (hepatitis), which can also manifest itself as jaundice, whereby the skin and eyes turn a yellowish colour, urine is brown and the stools noticeably light in colour.

In two thirds of those infected the immune system defends itself swiftly and successfully against the hepatitis B virus, and the disease takes its course without any symptoms, or with mild symptoms such as loss of appetite, stomach ache, vomiting, tiredness or fever. Only in one third of cases does jaundice develop. The symptoms usually pass and the infection leads to lifelong immunity. In rare cases — mainly in babies or people with a weakened immune system — it can lead to acute and fatal liver failure.

In 2–4% of infected adolescents and adults, the liver inflammation becomes chronic. Although patients with this complaint may feel healthy, they can infect others with hepatitis B. In roughly one quarter of virus-carriers chronic hepatitis develops, which leads — in a quarter of such cases in turn — to cirrhosis of the liver, and sometimes to liver cancer, both of which are often fatal.

According to research literature, the overall death rate from hepatitis B is less than 1% of all hepatitis B infections.[98] Together with other northern and western European countries the number of cases of hepatitis B in the UK is relatively low. Hepatitis B cases are much more frequent in third-world countries and endemic in certain populations such as Hong Kong, due to lifestyle elements.

Other types of hepatitis viruses can also cause chronic liver inflammations. The hepatitis C virus leads to chronic liver conditions more frequently than type B. These two illnesses often occur simultaneously, especially in drug addicts. There is no vaccination against hepatitis C. The hepatitis A virus is mainly transmitted from person to person, although it can also be transmitted through food and drink. The incubation period is between fifteen and forty days, and the symptoms are generally mild.

There is a vaccine against hepatitis A for at-risk groups, namely laboratory staff who work with the virus, haemophiliacs, travellers to high-risk areas and individuals who are at risk due to their sexual behaviour. The vaccine can be given in combination with hepatitis B.

The vaccine

Hepatitis B vaccines are produced by means of genetic engineering. They are dead vaccines, which do not contain the whole virus, only parts of the virus-membrane, as well as additional aluminium compounds. To get a good immune-system response, three to four vaccinations must be given by injection within a twelve-month period.

In the UK only high-risk groups are vaccinated: that is, medical and nursing or care staff; intravenous drug users; prison inmates; prostitutes; close family members of a carrier; infants born to mothers carrying the hepatitis B virus; haemophiliacs and their carers; patients with chronic renal failure (dialysis); morticians and other occupational risk groups; people in sexual contact with hepatitis B virus carriers. Since April 2000, all pregnant women in the UK are tested for Hepatitis B as part of routine antenatal screening.

Vaccination failure and side effects

Even following three successive vaccinations, sufficient protection from hepatitis B is only achieved in 90–95% of those vaccinated. In healthy young adults, children and newborn babies the response rate to the vaccine is almost 100%. There is accumulating evidence to show that there is no need for boosters once the person is protected.[99] After vaccination the response to it, and its protective effect, should be checked, so that people may not wrongly believe themselves to be safe, and fail to take other protective measures.

In up to 30% of those vaccinated, vaccination itself leads to local reactions such as pain at the injection site, and to fever in 6% of cases. In rare cases, strong allergic reactions can develop after vaccination. Temporary joint pain and joint swelling, as well as a rash have also been reported as rare complications.

Recommendations and considerations

In the UK the present official vaccination programme only recommends vaccinating the risk groups listed above.

However, there are considerations to include the hepatitis B vaccination into the childhood vaccination programme in the future.

The decision to vaccinate or not is an individual one. The risk factors of the disease have to be weighed against the potential adverse effects of the vaccination. Together with other protective measures — such as the use of condoms, gloves, clean needles etc. — the selective immunization policy seems to be successful in reducing the number of cases. The additional protective measures can also protect against other infections such as HIV or other forms of hepatitis.

Flu (influenza)

The illness

From a medical point of view, only those illnesses caused by the influenza virus are termed *flu*, as opposed to *gastric influenza* or colds. There are three types of influenza virus (A, B and C), of which only type A can be dangerous, and which are primarily active in the winter months. The type A virus, in particular, has thousands of variants, which can change from year to year. It often spreads in 'flu-waves' across the globe.

Infection occurs via exhaled or coughed droplets, but only half of those infected actually fall ill. The immune system of others is able to keep the viruses in check. Influenza breaks out suddenly in a person, accompanied by loss of appetite, high temperature, shivering, headache and muscle pain. It is usually over in a week, although convalescence can last several weeks. Flu can lead to a whole series of complications such as middle-ear infections, sinusitis, chest infections or heart muscle inflammation (myocarditis). In those already suffering from chronic heart or lung disease and in the elderly, in particular, it can lead to pneumonia, which is often fatal. Even in a winter with a low incidence of the virus, 3000–4000 deaths may be attributed to influenza.

The vaccine

Flu vaccines have been around for several years. They are inactivated vaccines and are prepared each year according to the advice of the World Health Organization (WHO), which recommends which strains should be included. Influenza vaccination should be repeated each year with the appropriate, approved vaccine.

The vaccine is injected into subcutaneous fatty tissue or into muscle, and is effective after about two weeks. Vaccination is currently recommended for everybody over sixty-five years of age and also for all people over six months of age who are part of a high-risk group: asthmatics, diabetics, people suffering from Chronic Obstructive Pulmonary Disease (COPD), chronic heart disease, chronic kidney disease and immune-suppression illnesses, as well as people who live in residential homes. Healthcare workers are also offered the vaccine.

Women in the first three months of pregnancy should not be vaccinated against flu, nor should babies under the age of six months or people with an allergy to chicken protein. People who may have already been infected with a flu virus should be cautious about vaccination. The influenza vaccine is prepared from dead, highly-purified viruses grown in hens' eggs. Each year the vaccine contains components of virus strains related to those considered most likely to be circulating during the forthcoming winter. There are several vaccines that protect against different strains of influenza. Some of the ones currently available in the UK contain thiomersal and others don't (see page 94).

Vaccination failure and side effects

70–90% of healthy people respond to the vaccine by forming antibodies, whose protective effect lasts for a year at most. In older people, who are particularly at risk, the vaccination only elicits a defensive reaction in about half, and the protective effect also lasts for considerably less time, possibly only four months.[100] In addition, vaccination does not protect against *flu-type* illnesses, only against the influenza variants contained in the vaccine. If virus-types other than those experts have predicted and used in the vaccine appear, the vaccine can be largely ineffective, as was the case in Switzerland during the flu epidemic of 1997/98.[101]

Vaccination leads to temporary swelling at the injection site in a third of vaccinated people. Serious complications from flu vaccination are few and so far unconfirmed.

Recommendations and considerations

There are two arguments against immunization in relation to the indirect side effects of flu vaccination:

— Having had a feverish illness such as flu could provide the immune system with a better ability to cope with severe illness later on, thereby improving the overall health of the population. This, of course, does not account for already chronic and seriously ill patients.

— Flu clearly decreases the risk of getting skin cancer (melanoma). A similar link has been described with other cancer types (see the chapter: 'Vaccinations are not natural infections' page 32).[102]

Swine flu

The illness

Influenza A (H1N1), also called swine flu, is a strain of influenza endemic in pigs. This was possibly related to the flu outbreak in 1918, which caused more then fifty million deaths worldwide, although this is not certain. In 1976 there was an outbreak of swine flu in the US. A vaccination programme was started, and approximately 50 million people were vaccinated. This vaccination was associated with numerous cases of Guillain-Barré Syndrome, a paralysing neuromuscular disorder, and resulted in twenty-five deaths, more than caused by the disease.

Swine flu became pandemic again in 2009 and, at the time of writing, had caused the deaths of 1000 people worldwide. The death rate stands at 0.34 %, similar to that of annual flu. It is feared that more than one third of the population will be affected.

Symptoms of swine flu are high temperature, above 38°C, headaches, runny nose, sore throat, cough, vomiting and painful limbs and lethargy.

The groups most at risk are pregnant woman, people with chronic diseases of the heart, liver, lungs, kidneys or neuralgic diseases, people with diabetes, suppressed immune systems (for example due to cancer or HIV) and children. It is thought that people above sixty-five will have some protection against it.

The most common causes of death are respiratory failure, pneumonia, high fever and dehydration. The disease is spread through coughing, sneezing and touching something with the virus on it. It is most contagious during the first five days of the illness, but with children it can stay contagious for up to ten days.

The vaccine

The vaccine programme was started in the UK in October 2009, with priority going to the groups of people mentioned above, who were most vulnerable to serious illness from swine flu. It has also been offered to healthcare professionals and people living with someone whose immune system is compromised (for example, people with cancer or HIV).

There are two available vaccines, Pandemrix and Celvapan. The Pandemrix vaccine only requires one dose and the Celvapan vaccine requires two doses, three weeks apart. Pandemrix is being offered to pregnant women, and means they will be protected more quickly than from Celvapan, which requires two doses.[103]

Children aged between six months and five years are also being offered the vaccine in two doses, three weeks apart. The vaccines do not provide protection for babies under six months. At the time of writing, the decision on whether to vaccinate the wider population was dependant on how the pandemic evolves.

One of the vaccines licensed in the UK, Pandemrix, is not suitable for people with an allergy to eggs, but the other, Celvapan, is suitable. Pandemrix contains thiomersal. Official guidelines state that there is no evidence of risk from thiomersal in vaccines, including for children, pregnant women and their offspring (see page 18).

Vaccination failure and side effects

As the swine flu vaccines discussed here are an exact match to the swine flu strain that was circulating at the time of writing, they should give at least 70–80% protection against the virus. As flu vaccines vary each year according to the most prevalent strains of influenza at the time, the insertion of the H1N1 strain into the vaccine should not substantially affect the safety of the vaccine; it should be as safe as standard seasonal flu vaccines. But, as with any new vaccine, rare side effects cannot be identified or ruled out until the vaccine has been used by the wider population in general.[104]

The Pandemrix vaccine should not be given to people with an allergy to eggs, but the Celvapan vaccine is not prepared using eggs.[105]

Recommendations and considerations

It is clear that this will be a pandemic. For most people the illness will be like normal flu. But the risk of complications is greater for people with other health problems and pregnant women. Also young people and children are at more risk, and you should consider how your family and work will cope if you (and the people around you) are ill with this flu.

Some pregnant women may feel cautious about having the vaccine, but they are also particularly at risk from developing serious illness. The seasonal flu vaccine has been given to millions of pregnant women at all stages of their pregnancy with no reported safety concerns.

It is clear that the element of fear plays a major part in a pandemic, and it is interesting that not everybody will fall ill. The question is if a healthy hygienic life, with regular hand-washing, cleaning, healthy food and sufficient time for inner reflection, would not offer some protection, but of course no conclusive information is available on this.

Chickenpox (varicella)

The illness

Chickenpox is a highly infectious viral illness. Most people will have had chickenpox as a mild illness during childhood. It is transmitted through droplets in the air, and presents itself mostly as an itchy rash of fluid-filled blisters, which cover the whole body. It is often associated with malaise and mild fever. The severity of illness increases with age. Pneumonia is a potentially serious, but rare, complication. A person suffering from chickenpox is infectious till the last blister has dried (scabbed over).

There are about twenty-five deaths from chickenpox each year, mainly adults. The chickenpox virus can remain dormant in the nervous system and be re-activated to cause shingles *(herpes zoster)* later in life. Shingles appears as a painful rash and can lead to post-herpetic neuralgia, a chronic pain syndrome. There are one hundred deaths a year from shingles.[106]

There is a specific concern for pregnant women. Varicella during the first twenty weeks of pregnancy can lead to congenital varicella syndrome, though the risk is less than 1%. This can cause shortened limbs, skin scars, brain damage and cataracts. Another concern is if a pregnant mother contracts chickenpox close to the birth, as chickenpox in a newborn can be fatal. Passive immunization (by injection) with immunoglobulins might be appropriate to use in those situations.

The vaccine

The vaccine contains live attenuated *varicella zoster* virus. It is given as two doses, separated by at least six weeks. It does not produce maximum immunity against chickenpox infection until about six weeks after the second dose. There is no evidence to suggest that further booster doses are needed. It is contra-indicated in people who have Acquired Immune Deficiency Syndrome (AIDS), or individuals receiving immune-suppressive therapy.[107] The general contra-indications to vaccines also apply (see page 98–99).

Its use is currently restricted to specific circumstances, and is not included in the childhood immunization programme. Chickenpox in adults can be much more serious than chickenpox in children, so it is offered to adults and adolescents aged thirteen years and over who have not already had chickenpox. It is also recommended for healthcare workers.

General Considerations Before Immunization

Before making a decision, make sure you have all the information you need, and take your time. Vaccinations are not usually urgent.

— There is no such thing as absolute safety. An illness can lead to severe complications and ensuing damage, but this cannot be excluded in the case of vaccination either.

— Especially in the case of children, the official vaccination programme represents a multitude of different immunizations within a short period of time at a very young age. This programme currently advised in the UK is only a recommendation and is not obligatory.

— Weigh up the usefulness and risks of vaccination against the risks and possible usefulness of an illness, both for yourself and your child.

— For small children it might be better not to start vaccinations too early, since their immune and nervous systems are still developing. One could argue that in the cases of Hib, meningitis C and whooping cough, that there is an urgency to vaccinate a child as young as possible. There is no urgency for any other of the vaccinations to be given to young babies, but unfortunately, the whooping cough vaccine is not available as a single vaccine.

— Vaccination protection can fade with time, so make sure you have a booster when it is due, and also check the immunity status for German measles when girls enter puberty.

— Caution is recommended for pregnant women.

— Caution is recommended if you suffer from an acute illness.

— Where possible ask for vaccines without mercury-based thiomersal.

— In the case of combined vaccines, try to make sure that you don't receive unnecessary vaccines for diseases against which you are already protected (either by previous vaccination or natural immunity).

— Stand up for your personal vaccination decision, but consider the consequences of confrontation with health professionals; they act according to their best knowledge. You have made such decisions based on your best knowledge and conscience.

— Consult your doctor if severe side effects occur following vaccinations, or if side effects continue for more than two days. Discuss with your doctor the need for reporting any occurring side effects (e.g. Yellow Card Scheme in the UK, or VAERS programme in the US).

Current UK Childhood Vaccination Schedule

Routine childhood immunization programme in 2009[108]

Disease (vaccine)	Comment	Age
Diphtheria, tetanus, pertussis, polio and Hib (DTaP/IPV/Hib combined)	primary course (3 doses)	2 months 3 months 4 months
Pneumococcal infection (PCV)	3 doses	2 months 4 months 13 months
Meningitis C (MenC)	primary course (2 doses)	3 months 4 months
Hib and meningitis C (Hib/MenC combined)	booster	12 months
Measles, mumps and rubella (MMR combined)	2 doses	13 months 3 yrs 4 mths to 5 years
Diphtheria, tetanus, pertussis and polio (DTaP/IPV combined)	booster	3 yrs 4 mths to 5 years
Diphtheria, tetanus and polio (Td/IPV combined)	booster	13–18 years
Human papillomavirus (HPV)	3 doses over 6 months	12–13 years

References

1 Dr Hoppeler, circa 1900, quoted in: *Pharma Information: Dossier Gesundheit,* issue 3, July 1996, 'Die Impfung hat Geburtstag'

2 Dr Henderson et al.: 'Smallpox and Vaccinia' in: S. Plotkin, E. Mortimer: *Vaccines.* Saunders 1994, p. 13–40; Bulletin of World Health Organization 1975; 52: 209–22; *British Medical Journal* 1995, 310: 62

3 L. Sagan: *Die Gesundheit der Nationen — Die eigentlichen Ursachen von Gesundheit und Krankheit im Weltvergleich,* Rowohlt, Hamburg 1992

4 L. Sagan. See note 3

5 P. Cotton: 'Das CDC wird bald fünfzig sein', in: *JAMA Schweiz,* no. 10, October 1990, p. 429 f.

6 P. Klein: 'Die Krux mit den Impfnebenwirkungen', in: B. Gruber, R. Heimann, P. Jenni et al.: *Impfen, Routine oder Individualization, Eine Standortbestimmung aus hausärztlicher Sicht,* Bern 199, p. 67

7 A. Zott: 'Für und Wider von multikomponenten Impfstoffen', in: *Deutsches Bundesgesundheitsblatt,* no. 12, 1997, p. 498–501

8 W. Huber: 'Nebenwirkungen der Impfstoff-Additive Aluminium-Hydroxid und Thimersal am Beispiel des Impfstoffs gegen Hepatitis B', in: *Oekoskop,* no. 1, 1995

9 H. Bedford, D. Elliman: *Childhood Immunisation: The Facts,* Health Promotion, England 2001

10 D. Primarolo: 'Daily Hansard, Column 1366W', from: www.parliament.uk, England 26 July 2007

11 P. F. King, D. P. Perl, L, M. Brieree, et al.: ' Selective accumulation of aluminium and iron in the neurofibrillarytangles of Alzheimer's disease', in: *Annals of Neurology,* 1992; 31: 286–92

12 E. von Mutius et al.: 'Prevalence of asthma and allergic disorders among children in United Germany: a descriptive comparison', in: *British Journal of Medicine,* no. 305, 1992, p.

1395–1399

13 J. Alm et al.: 'Atopy in children of families with an anthroposophic lifestyle', in: *The Lancet*, no. 353, 1998, p. 1485–1488

14 S. Shaheen et al.: 'Measles and atopy in Guinea Bissau', in: *The Lancet*, no. 347, 1996, p. 1792–1794

15 Cf. U. Koch: *Impfen im Kindes- und Erwachsenenalter, Ein kritischer Ratgeber aus homöopathischer Sicht*, Schriftenreihe von Natur und Medizin e.V., Veronica Carstens, 2nd edition, Bonn 1997, p. 35–39

16 B. Spring: 'Zeitpunkt der Impfung und Impfabstände', in: B. Gruber, R. Heimann, P. Jenni et al., see note 6

17 P. Klein, H.U. Albonico: *Der individuelle Impfentscheid*, Merkblatt der Arbeitsgruppe für differenzierte Impfungen, Bern, October 2001

18 P. Farrington et al.: 'A new method for active surveillance of adverse effects from diphtheria/tetanus/pertussis and measles/mumps/rubella vaccines', in: *The Lancet*, no. 345, 1995, p. 567–569

19 Center for Disease Control (CDC): Adverse Events following Immunisation — *Surveillance Report 1989*, CDC/US Department of Health and Human Services, Atlanta 1989, p. 6

20 J. Classen, D. Classen: 'Hemophilus vaccine and increased IDDM, causal relationship likely', in: *British Medical Journal*, no. 319, 1999, p. 1133

21 H. von Zimmermann: 'Masernschutzimpfung einschränken!' in *Pädiatrische Praxis*, no. 34, 1986/87, p.587–593

22 H. L. Coulter: *Vaccination, Social Violence and Criminality, The Medical Assault on the American Brain*, North Atlantic Books, Berkeley Ca. 1990

23 A. J. Wakefield et al.: 'Ileal-lymphoid nodular hyperplasmia, nonspecific colitis and pervasive developmental disorder in children', in: *The Lancet*, no. 351, 1998, p. 637–641; O. Sheils & J. J. O'Leary et al. (2002); Abstract (No 20) presented at Pathological Society of Great Britain and Ireland, www.pathsoc.org.uk

24 M. Glöckler, W. Goebel: *A Guide to Child Health*, Floris Books, 2003. p.129f.

25 Dr W. Havinga: 'Is Your Body a Mystery?', www.

everydaymedicine.com, 2000

26 M. Glöckler, W. Goebel: see note 24, p.140f.

27 B. Gruber, R. Wegmüller: 'Krankheitskonzepte', in: B. Gruber, R. Heimann, P. Jenni et al., see note 6, p. 70

28 M. Glöckler, W. Goebel: note 24, Chapter 9, pp.139–148

29 H. U. Albonico: *Gewaltige Medizin, Fragen eines Hausarztes zur Immunologie, zu den Impfungen gegen Kinderkrankeheiten, zu AIDS and zur Gentechnologie,* Verlag Paul Haupt, 2nd edition, Berne, Stuttgart, Vienna 1998, p. 43, 51f.

30 H. M. Stellmann: *Kinderkrankheiten natürlich behandeln,* Gräfe und Unzer, 4th edition, Munich 1993, p. 79

31 I. Duffell. E. J. Epidemiol Community Health 2001; 55: 685–686

32 E. von Mutius: *Epidemiologie des Asthma Bronchiale im Kindesalter. Pneumologie.* 1997; 51: 949–61

33 *Journal of Paediatrics* 1986, 108, p. 671–76

34 Cf. R.A. Lawrence: *Breastfeeding, A guide for the medical profession,* 5th edition, Mosby 1999

35 R. Schmidt: 'Krebs und Infektionskrankheiten', in: *Medizinische Klinik,* no. 43, 1910, p. 1630–1633

36 Cf. U. Abel: ' Infekthäufigkeit und Krebsrisiko', in: *Deutsche medizinische Wochenschrift,* no. 111, 1986, p. 1978–1981

37 McGowan et al.: 'The woman at risk of developing ovarian cancer', in: *Gynaecological Oncology,* no. 7, 1979, p. 325–344

38 H. U. Albonico et al.: 'Febrile infectious childhood diseases in the history of cancer patients and matched controls', in: *Medical Hypotheses,* no. 51, 1988, p. 315–320

39 J. Kesselring: 'Zur Pathogenese der Multiplen Sklerose', in: *Schweizerische medizinische Wochenschrift,* no. 20, 1990, p. 1083–1090

40 The MMR Discussion Pack, NHS Scotland

41 National Vaccine Advisory Committee USA: *The Measles Epidemic,* JAMA, 1991, p. 266

42 Cf. CDC: 'Measles Outbreak — Netherlands', April 1999–January 2000, in: *MMWR,* no. 14, April 2000, p. 299–303

43 J. Lederberg: 'Emerging viruses — emerging threat', in:

Science, no. 247, 1990, p. 279–280

44 P. Klein, H.U. Albonico: *Der individuelle Impfentscheid.* See note 17

45 H. Sternberger: 'Pneumokokken-Impfung immer wichtiger — Diese Bakterien besetzen die von Hämophilus befreiten Nischen', in *Ärzte-Woche,* April 1996

46 M. Koskiniemi: 'Epidemiology of Encephalitis in children: A Prospective Multicentre Study', *Eur J Paediatric.* 1997; 156: 541–5

47 M. Müller: 'Die M+M+R-Impfkampagne des Bundes auf dem juristischen Prüfstand', in: *Scweizerische Ärztezeitung,* no. 10, 1994, p. 385–390

48 H. Bedford, D. Elliman. See note 9

49 W. Goebel, M. Glöckler. See note 24, p. 225 ff.

50 H. Bedford, D. Elliman. See note 9; Centre for Disease Control, Diphtheria epidemic — new independent states of former Soviet Union, 1990-1994, *Morbidity and Mortality,* weekly report, 1995; 44(10); 177–81

51 N. T. Begg, V. Balraj: ' Diphtheria: are we ready for it?', in: *Archives of Disease in Childhood,* 1995; 73: 568–72

52 NHS: 'Tetanus Cases 1984-2003', from: www.immunisation. nhs.uk/Vaccines/DTaP_IPV_Hib/The_diseases/Tetanus/ Tetanus_Cases_1984-2003, 2008

53 World Health Organization: 'Global Immunization Coverage', from: http://www.who.int/immunization_monitoring, October 2009

54 NHS: 'Preventing tetanus', from: www.nhs.uk/Conditions/ Tetanus/Pages/Prevention, August 2009

55 Department of Health: *Immunisation against Infectious Diseases,* 1996

56 K. Stehr: *Schutzimpfung gegen Pertussis,* Medizinische Verlagsbuchhandlung, Marburg/Lahn, 1985

57 H. Bedford, D. Elliman. See note 9

58 V. Jenni: 'Pertussis', in: B. Gruber, R. Heimann, P. Jenni et al. See note 6, p. 23.

59 H. Bedford et al: 'National follow-up of Haemophilus influenza meningitis', letter from: *Archives of Disease in Childhood* 1993; 69: 711–12

60 H. Bedford, D. Elliman. See note 9

61 M. Karvonene et al: 'Association between type 1 diabetes and Haemophilus influenzae type b vaccination: birth cohort study', in: *British Medical Journal*, no. 318, 1999, p. 1169–1172

62 M. Karvonene et al: 'Diabetes mellitus nach Impfung gegen H. Influenzae Typ B (HiB-Vaccinol U.A.)', in: *arznei-telegramm*, no. 11, 1999, p. 120

63 H. Bedford, D. Elliman. See note 9.

64 J. Ward: 'Haemophilus Influenzae Vaccines', in: S. Plotkin, E. Mortimer. See note 2, p. 344–346

65 Department of Health. See note 55

66 Ibid.

67 Chief Medical Officer: Update 27.

68 Department of Health. See note 55

70 BAG: 'Neue Empfehlungen zur Poliomyelitisimpfung', in: *BAG Bulletin*, no. 43, 25 October 1999, p. 809

71 L.K. Pickering: 'Report of the Committee on Infectious Diseases, 2000', American Academy of Pediatrics, Illinois 2000

72 H. U. Albonico: 'Argumente gegen die routinemässige Mumpsimpfung', in: *Sozial und Präventivmedizin*, no. 40, 1995, p. 116–123

73 P. Klein: 'Masern', in: B. Gruber, R. Heimann, P. Jenni et al. See note 6, p. 33

74 A. Lienhard: *Impfen: ein Ratgeber*, Almada Verlag Winterthur 1998, p.57

75 NHS Scotland: 'MMR fact sheet No. 1'

76 Public Health Laboratory Service: www.phls.co.uk, accessed 19 October 2002

77 NHS: 'Measles "Surge" Q&A', www.nhs.uk/news/2008/11november/pages/measlessurgeqa, November 2008

78 NHS Scotland: 'MMR fact sheet No. 1'

79 Robert Koch Institut: 'Nationales Referenzzentrum für Masern, Mumps und Röteln', in *Epidemiologisches Bulletin*, no. 46, 1996, p. 318

80 National Vaccine Advisory Committee USA. See note 41, p. 266

81 NHS Scotland: 'Measles Fact sheet No.1'

82 H. U. Albonico et al.: 'Schweizerische Impfkampagne gegen Masern, Mumps und Röteln — Ärztliche Bedenken zur Ausrottungs-Strategie', in: Schweizerische *Zeitschrift für GanzheitsMedizin* 1994, no. 1, p. 38–41, and no. 2, p. 68–73

83 Ärztegruppe für differenzierte MMR-Impfungen (ed.): *Masern, Mumps und Röteln-Impfungen: Warum die Eltern mitentscheiden sollen*, 4th enlarged edition, Bern 1994, p.2

84 Department of Health: *Protecting Women against Rubella*, September 2003.

85 Ibid.

86 WHO Copenhagen: *Expanded Programme on Immunisation — Report of the Meeting of National Programme Managers 1989*, Copenhagen 1989, UNO

87 P. Stohrer-Draxl et al.: 'Masern, Mumps und Röteln: Durchimpfungsrate und Seroprävalenz bei 8. Klässlern in acht verschiedenen Orten der Schweiz 1995/96', in: *Praxis*, no. 88, 1999, p. 1069–1077

88 H. U. Albonico et al., 1994. See note 82, p. 70f.

89 BMJ Publishing Group: Clinical Evidence, June 2001

90 Dr P. Owen: 'Cervical cancer', from: www.netdoctor.co.uk/diseases/facts/cervicalcancer, Netdoctor, May 2005

91 NHS: 'About the HPV vaccine', from: www.immunisation.nhs.uk/Vaccines/HPV/About_the_HPV_vaccine, 2008

92 Netdoctor: 'Gardasil (HPV vaccine)', from: http://www.netdoctor.co.uk/medicines/100003034.html, December 2008

93 Daily Mail: 'Concerns over safety of cervical cancer vaccine after 1300 girls experience adverse side-effects', from: www.dailymail.co.uk/health/article-1160516/Paralysis-epilepsy-blurred-vision-1-300-girls-reaction-cervical-cancer-vaccine.html, March 2009

94 NHS: 'Having the vaccination', from: http://www.immunisation.nhs.uk/Vaccines/HPV/Having_the_vaccination, 2008

95 World Health Organisation: '2009 Update Tuberculosis Facts', from: www.who.int/tb/publications/2009/tbfactsheet_2009update_one_page.pdf, 2009

96 Department of Health. See note 55

97 British Medical Association and Royal Pharmaceutical society of Great Britain: *British National Formula*, September 2003

98 S. Krugmann et al.: 'Hepatitis B Vaccine', in: S. Plotkin, E. Mortimer. See note 2, p. 420

99 European Consensus Group on Hepatitis B Immunity, 2000

100 A. Lienhard. See note 74, p. 107

101 Bundesamt für Gesundheit: 'Grippeepidemiologie 1997/98 und Impfstoffzumsammensetzung 1998/99', in: *BAG-Bulletin*, no. 40, 1998, p.34

102 K. Kömel et al.: 'Infections and melanoma risk', in: *Melanoma Research*, no. 9, 1999, p.511–519

103 Department of Health: 'Swine Flu and Pregnancy', from: www.dh.gov.uk/prod_consum_dh/groups/dh_digitalassets/@dh/@en/documents/digitalasset/dh_108154.pdf, November 2009

104 NHS: 'Information on the swine flu vaccine', from: www.nhs.uk/conditions/pandemic-flu/pages/vaccine, December 2009

105 Department of Health: 'Swine flu vaccination: what you need to know', from: www.nhs.uk/Conditions/pandemic-flu/Documents/SF%20vaccination%20leaflet_web.pdf, October 2009

106 H. Bedford, D. Elliman. See note 9

107 British Medical Association and Royal Pharmaceutical society of Great Britain. See note 97

108 NHS: 'Routine childhood immunisation programme in 2009', from: www.immunisation.nhs.uk/Immunisation_Schedule, 2008

Further Reading

Books

Bedford, Helen and Elliman, David, *Childhood Immunisation: the Facts*, Health Promotion England, 2001.

Glöckler, M. and Goebel, W., *A Guide to Child Health*, Floris Books, 2003.

Goebel, Dr W., *Schutzimpfungen selbst verantwortet*, Verlag Freies Geistesleben, 2002.

Halvorsen Richard, *The Truth About Vaccines: Making the Right Decision for Your Child*, Gibson Square Books Ltd, 2009.

Joint Committee on Vaccination and Immunisation, *Immunisation and Infectious disease*, Department of Health, 2006.

Murphy, Christine, *The Vaccination Dilemma*, Lantern Books, 2002.

Research Publications

S. J. Alm et al., 'Atopy in children of families with an anthroposophic lifestyle,' *The Lancet*, 1 May 1999, Vol. 353, No. 9163, pages 1485–1488

Websites

www.doh.gov.uk Department of Health

www.immunisation.nhs.uk and www.immunisation.org.uk NHS immunization websites

www.nhs.uk/Conditions/Immunisations-childhood NHS direct

www.netdoctor.co.uk An informative medical website, recommended by GPs

www.hpa.org.uk Health Protection Agency

www.mhra.gov.uk Medicines and Healthcare products Regulatory Agency (MHRA)

www.publichealth.hscni.net Public Health Agency

www.informedparent.co.uk 'The Informed Parent'

www.jabs.org.uk 'JABS' (Justice, Awareness & Basic Support)

www.mmrthefacts.nhs.uk further information on the MMR vaccine

www.ahasc.org.uk Anthroposophic Health and Social Care

Index